IF I STOP SMOKING NOW WILL THE CANCER GO AWAY?

Jane Stanhope

This is a story. This is a true story.

The names, characters, places and incidents have been changed in order to protect identities where appropriate.

Should there be any resemblance to an actual person, living or dead, business establishments, events or locales it is entirely coincidental.

IF I STOP SMOKING NOW

WILL THE CANCER GO AWAY?

Published by Jane Stanhope

Copyright © 2016 by Jane Stanhope

Cover Art by Jane Stanhope

Chapter ONE

I hate this purse! I can't find a freaking thing in it! It's beautiful and I paid more than two-hundred-fifty dollars for the thing when it was on sale. Everybody compliments the stupid thing. And I love the way it looks! But I hate it! It's too complicated for me. I thought because it has so many pockets and compartments inside of it, that I would be able to organize my stuff. I thought I could have one compartment for makeup and one for keys and one for money. I thought I would have one special place for everything and then I would always know where my stuff was. But it isn't working! The problem is that I can never remember which compartment is for which thing. And to make it even worse, I'm always too busy to pay attention to the compartments and the original compartment plan. I get busy and I just throw things back into the beautiful purse that it feels like I paid a fortune for. So now when I'm searching for something; that thing that I'm looking for can literally be anywhere inside of this purse! I can't for the life of me ever find a thing in it!

"Where the hell is that stupid phone?!" This is the one thing that for some reason is the most impossible to find! It's the one thing that gets buried deeper and deeper within the many hidden caves and compartments of my beautiful dark burgundy patent leather giant freaking purse! It's the one thing that requires me to have a huge sense of urgency for when I have to find it. It's the one thing that demands my time! And when these demands are being made I only have so much time to find it. Because if I don't find it I will most assuredly miss the call which most assuredly would have presented me with something extremely important and life changing! And it won't stop ringing! And I actually shouldn't even call it ringing. It's more like screaming! It's some sort of song that all of the young people like and I can't hear the words. It's on the radio all day long apparently. I don't even know the name of it. My daughter put it on my phone and I don't know how to get it off of it. I do know that I hate it! And right now that stupid ring-song seems to be causing the walls and rooftop of the off-season rental cottage that I'm stuck in for the time being to vibrate with every pulsating beat of its foolish melody! It's getting louder and louder as I burrow deeper and deeper into my beautiful purse!

"GOD DAMMIT!" I just know I'll never get to it in time. But the fact that it's getting louder is a good sign. I'm getting closer to it! Close enough that I'm holding the purse as wide open as I possibly can and I've shoved my face half-way into the freaking thing to try and catch a glimpse of the light that the cell-phone is most assuredly shining, as it continues to scream at the top of its tiny cell phone lungs! I swear to Christ I'm just going to dump the entire freaking thing out and onto the floor! And then I'm going to start throwing all of my makeup, money, credit cards, papers, tissues, lotions and a tiny package of crackers across the room as I explode with a ginormous rage which causes complete destruction of the contents within the deep burgundy patent leather giant freaking purse!

"Shit! There it is!" Finally I snatch my phone from its hiding spot and throw my beautiful purse back into the kitchen chair it quietly rested on before the horrific ring-singing started.

"Hello?" I'm out of breath. Holy crap! I feel like I just ran a freaking marathon.

"Jane?"

"Yes." Who is this? I don't know the number that's shown up on my cell-phone. I'm panting as I plop myself onto the ugly sofa in the tiny living room. I hate that there's no caller ID on cell-phones. More than half of the calls I receive pop through as 'unknown' and sometimes 'private' and the other half are just a jumble of numbers that I can't remember. Why don't we have the technology yet that will allow me to do a better screening of the calls coming in? Or do we and my phone just sucks? When I was ten years old I remembered everybody's number but since then I've become dependent on technology and now I remember absolutely nothing!

"This is Brad from the Orthopedic Center. We have the results from your MRI."

"Oh, hello Brad." I knew I recognized the number. I take a nice deep breath and slowly blow it back out. It's weird that he's just 'Brad'. Why isn't he 'Doctor Something'? I think he's working towards becoming a doctor but he's not quite there yet. That's probably why he's just 'Brad'.

"We do see some tendonitis in your shoulder and there are

some calcifications. Fortunately there is no tearing of the rotator cuff, though." He sounds so serious. This is good news isn't it? Why isn't he happy for me? Why isn't he more pleasant sounding? I mean I know 'Brad' doesn't even know me and he only met me a couple of weeks ago when I finally caved in to the excruciating pain and dragged myself and my dead shoulder, which therefore includes my arm, into the Orthopedic Center. And of course I had brought Albert with me for the appointment.

The office was so sunny and clean. The people that worked behind the counters and through the glass all smiled and welcomed us to the office. Both Albert and I were immediately comfortable in our surroundings. Everybody seemed so nice. Being new to the area not only do we find ourselves looking at locations but we also find ourselves looking for people. We want to be near people that are nice to us. We want to feel welcome. And when we enter a new place, whether it's an office or a restaurant, we take note of the genuine nature of the people that are already there. And we wonder which community they live in. There's only one way to find the answers to our questions, so that's when the talking begins. Mostly from Albert.

Years ago we lived here when I transferred from Maine to New Hampshire due to my job with a giant big retail store. And we liked living here back then so we were excited when we got the news that I was being transferred back to the Granite State again due to my current job with a different company but nonetheless another giant big retail store. Back to a State that has communities full of people that are actually nice. I wondered if any of the people we were meeting at the Orthopedic Center would actually become some of the people we would come to know in the community that we would come to live in.

After checking in we were instructed to sit in the waiting room which already had a dozen patients in it. The room was quiet and smelled as if a maintenance man had just come through and disinfected the entire place with a concoction of lemons and pine. Albert and I chose a couple of chairs near the windows and positioned ourselves as best we could. The chairs were pretty to look at but unbelievably uncomfortable. I sat straight up and flipped through the many pages of repetitive paperwork that the nice ladies at the greeting window gave me.

Albert leaned back and suddenly began to hum to the music that piped through an impressive speaker system in the crisp white tiled ceiling. At first I thought he was only going to hum for a split second as he settled. Then he would begin to stare at the many people in the waiting room. Albert and I both love to watch people so I assumed he would settle and begin the task of staring and figuring out who everybody was and exactly what they were doing here, but Albert didn't stop humming. He actually seemed to be enjoying the music and began to hum even louder. And as he continued to hum he began to bob his head up and down. And the waiting room which had been completely quiet when we first entered began to shift. Nobody was talking. Everybody was minding their own business and quietly turning pages of magazines or books. But now as they quietly sat and read, they began to shuffle. They twisted in their chairs and they crinkled the pages of the magazines loudly. All of them could obviously hear him. It was as if he was screaming and yelping for the entire room to stop what they were doing and 'JUST LOOK AT ME!' Albert didn't know, understand or care about the impact he was having and was completely oblivious to the fact that he was disturbing an entire room full of people. Maybe he just didn't see it? Regardless, Albert just kept humming. The song that initially embraced the waiting room people and offered them comfort as they politely held their place in line to see the nurses and doctors who'd promised to help them, was being taken away from them. The entire atmosphere of the quiet and comforting waiting room had changed. And the people in the waiting room were all staring at Albert with disdain.

And it's not like the two of us entering any facility/business/waiting room in the entire state of New Hampshire is not already enough reason to cause staring, given the fact that I'm as white as the driven snow and Albert is not; but does he have to demand even more attention? What is this burning desire that my husband seems to have to constantly be at the center of attention? Is it because he's one of eight children and he grew up having to misbehave in order to get the already strained attention from his mother or older siblings that were forced to watch and hopefully control him and his younger brothers and sisters while his mother was at work??

Casually I leaned toward Albert. "Will you please stop?" I'm whisper yelling as I glare into Albert's eyes.

"What?" Of course he doesn't whisper his response which causes the others in the waiting room to cross their brows even more as the staring continues. Three of the men in the waiting room folded their arms across their chest and two of the women changed the legs which they had crossed to the other side. And all of them shifted in the more than uncomfortable waiting room chairs.

I looked back down at the clipboard full of paperwork that I still had to complete and I began to fill in the many blanks as I shook my head back and forth with disgust for Albert. Approximately ten minutes later I finished and felt that enough time had probably passed; I thought perhaps that the 'others' in the waiting room had stopped staring at the show between me and Albert. I thought that perhaps they'd become used to the fact that Albert continued to bob his stupid head up and down to every beat of the once comforting music. I hoped that his ridiculous humming was close enough to the actual tone of the music that it had started to blend in with the actual music so perhaps wasn't as noticeable as when we first sat down. I was nervous when I quietly raised my head and began to stare back at the others.

'Phew! Thank God they're not staring at us!'

Directly across the room from where we sat was an elderly couple. They looked like farmers. The man was wearing a dark green canvas type work shirt and I noticed at least two layers of under-shirts peeking through the top collar area of the over-shirt. And over the top of the dark green canvas type work shirt he wore a wool vest that zipped up the front. His farmer hat was cream colored and it had sweat stains that ran all the way around the circumference of his head. He looked tired. Like maybe he had been up all night because whatever the reason that brought him into the doctor's office today was hurting him horribly. He reminded me of my grandfather except that he hadn't shaved. My grandfather shaved every morning. And he always smelled like Old Spice. The man sitting across the room didn't smell like my grandfather though. At least I don't think he did. By the looks of it, I'd say he smelled like hay or cut grass even though it was snowing outside. He probably smelled like the sweat that's staining the cream colored farmer's hat.

"Mr. Glenn?" One of the nurses from behind the tan wooden door walked into the waiting room and smiled as she held it open for Mr. Glenn.

His last name is Glenn? I wonder if he's related to that astronaut! He sort of looks like him!

The farmer and his wife stood up and it was immediately obvious why they were there. The elderly farmer clung to his wife's arm as he hobbled through the tan door with the smiling nurse.

"I'll bet a horse stepped on his foot." I leaned toward Albert and whispered.

"HA!" Albert and his explosive belly laugh caused nothing but more attention in our direction from the 'others' who were beginning to growl as they shifted yet again in the uncomfortable chairs. They had reached their level of saturation with Albert's humming, head bobbing and bursts of comment and laughter.

I angrily glared at him again. What the hell was I thinking about even talking to him? And perhaps the better question is, 'what the hell is wrong with him?' I really do think that perhaps his mental capacity seized still when he was a child and he will always and forever be stuck in 1970. Even though he gets older he cannot keep himself from battling for attention from his over-worked and frazzled mother. That's got to be it! Dammit, why didn't I just leave him at home? 'Home' meaning that stupid cottage that we're renting!

"Did you call Mary and schedule us to see more houses?" Suddenly Albert is talking to me as if we are the only two people in the room. Like he could care less if the 'others' are annoyed, interrupted or continuing to growl! What was he doing? He shouldn't be talking in public about anything that is going on in our lives! The others don't need to know any of our business! Why is he always so freaking loud?!

More angry staring on my part.

"What?" Again with the explosive need for attention.

Suddenly a little person walked into the waiting area. He was only about three and one half feet tall and he used crutches for help as he wriggled his way to an empty seat and struggled to get comfortable in it. His eyes were a piercing blue color and his cheek bones were well chiseled behind a beautiful blanket of satin skin. I imagined how attractive he would be if he were six feet tall and wondered if he was married. He must be. He's beautiful. When he noticed me staring at him he smiled; I nodded my head and smiled back.

Albert slowly began to lean in my direction and I could tell he wanted to say something.

Quickly I snapped my head toward Albert and cast him a glare which threatened to absolutely kill him right there in the middle of the waiting room full of witnesses. He immediately knew what my glare was screaming at him and began to laugh. My glare continued to burrow a hole right through Albert's brain as it screamed for him to shut the hell up and not even think for a minute that the word he wanted so badly to say would even come close to escaping his insensitive and ignorant lips! Slowly I shook my head back and forth and curled my lips to a snarl. Albert was desperately trying not to laugh and I could see tears welling up in his eyes. He reminded me of a dog I'd seen on the television.

This particular dog was an Australian Shepherd and he was notorious for stealing food items from the counter in his owner's kitchen. And his absolute favorite thing of all things to snatch, run away with, hide with and ultimately devour was cupcakes. On this particular television show that I watched, the family of the cupcake thieving dog had called in an expert to try and train the dog to stop the misbehaving habit. At one point the trainer had the owner of the dog prepare the most adorable cupcakes. They were yellow cake with pretty pink frosting and a host of colorful sprinkles over the top. Just seeing the cupcakes on the television, I could smell their warm yummy aroma and I myself wished I could just reach through the television screen and snatch one from the kitchen counter in the dog owner's home. And when the trainer attempted the ultimate test for the Australian Shepherd, he held a platter full of the delicious looking cupcakes right in the front of the pooch's nose. The look on the dog's face was hysterical! His glowing blue eyes were huge and fixated on the pink frosting with the host of colorful sprinkles. He slowly leaned his head to the left and continued to just stare at the cupcakes! His tongue was hanging out and he licked his lips in desperation while he never took his eyes away from the delectable prize! The trainer whisper-yelled some sort of noise that sounded like "check" over and over at the dog as the drooling continued. And as much as he wanted to, the dog never snatched one of the delectable cupcakes from the platter! Talk about self-control!

And that's Albert, right now! He's leaning his head to the left, his eyes are watering and he's slowly but assuredly forming that horrible word and he's starting to mouth it to me without even a hint of a whisper. But he knows me. He sees the look on my face and within my mind I'm screaming at him that strange whisper of a word that the trainer screamed at the Australian Shepherd: 'check…check!' He realizes that if I hear the sound of the first letter of that word, I will choke him out right here in the crisp white waiting room that's still playing the joyful music that he hummed and bobbed his head to when we first sat down! I wonder what the consequences were for the Australian Shepherd if he failed. I wonder if the dog knew.

"Jane?" The nurse is back and holding open the tan door for me to walk through.

"Mmmmm…" Albert stood up.

I snapped my head toward him with horrific anger and continued to approach the nurse and the open door. Albert is lucky that the first letter of the horrific word is an 'm' because he can easily claim that he's continuing to hum to the joyful music as I unjustly accuse him of being an insensitive jerk. As we walked through the door Albert exploded with laughter as I spun on my heels and punched him right in the side of his arm!

"Everything okay?" The nurse was giggling at the sight of us.

"It will be if you have a weapon I can borrow?" I was angry but I started laughing as well.

"What?" Now she was confused.

"Nothing." Albert and I both laughed out loud and disrupted the professional and quiet atmosphere of the hidden rooms behind the tan door that led to the quiet waiting room.

We followed the nurse's instructions and settled into another room, which truly is nothing more than a smaller version of the waiting room with fewer magazines and entertainment. The nurse smiled as she took my vital signs.

"Why are you here?" She continued to smile as she asked

the question.

"My shoulder hurts."

Two appointments, a series of x-rays and finally an MRI followed that initial morning when I had finally come to the conclusion that the pain in my shoulder probably indicated that I in fact had an injury that would require some sort of attention and HELP. I hate going to the doctor with a complaint which amounts to nothing more than a younger than I am professional explaining to me that 'at my age it is normal to have some arthritis, bursitis or tendonitis.' Why would I waste my money on an appointment that amounts to a complete stranger telling me that I'm freaking old? So that is why I never go to the doctor unless I'm completely positive that whatever is going on with me is beyond what I can handle by myself with over the counter drugs and research on the internet. And it is because I had reached this stage with the explosive pain in my right shoulder that I found myself sitting in that tiny second waiting room with crisp white ceiling tiles. That was the reason I began to cry when the nurse made me attempt to move my arm which hung practically lifeless at my side.

"We recommend a treatment program of Ultrasound Therapy, which should help to break up the calcifications that you have in your shoulder."

"Okay."

Brad still sounds so serious. This is the guy that we eventually met in the second room, the smaller waiting room with hardly any magazines, who talked to Albert for an hour after he completed the examination of my shoulder. And I swear to God the two of them are like long lost cousins or something; even though they look nothing alike. Brad actually looks like one of my cousins! In fact he looks exactly like my cousin. It's weird.

You know that eerie feeling when you meet somebody and you discover that everything in their life is parallel to your own? You both have a sister that's a Graphic Artist. You both grew up in a small town in Maine. You both collect antique school bells. And suddenly you feel like you're staring at yourself in a mirror which reflects the inner soul; not the skin. Well, that is what happened when Albert met Brad. That first appointment at the Orthopedic Center ended up taking a full hour and a half when it probably only needed to be twenty minutes. Albert and Brad couldn't stop talking.

"There was also something that showed up at the very edge of the scan. Sort of outside of the viewing area." Brad pauses.

"Oh okay. What was it?" What the hell is he talking about? Get back to the calcification things and how he's going to get rid of this freaking pain so I can start using my arm again. I have questions to ask him; like does the ultrasound stuff sort of zap it? Is it like an explosion in my arm when they do that? Will I need Novocain? Does it hurt?

"I'm not sure." He pauses again.

"So where do I go for the ultrasound stuff?" Get to the point Brad.

He clears his throat. "Right here at the Orthopedic Center."

"Should I just call for an appointment or is somebody going to call me?" I'm feeling anxious for some reason to get the solution going. Could be because I can't move my freaking arm!

"Somebody will call you." Pausing again. "I can give you the direct telephone number also in case you want to call."

"How long will the ultrasound thing take? Do I have to go just one time or more than that?" I'm scrambling through the kitchen drawer, at the seasonal rental cottage as I try to find a pen and scrap of paper.

More clearing of his throat. What the hell is wrong with him? "Well, it depends." Another pause. "Jane you're going to want to make an appointment with your primary care doctor for follow up."

"Follow up? Follow up for what?" I've moved onto drawer number three as I continue to scramble. Where the hell is a pen? Dammit! I think there's one in my freaking purse. Oh God, not the purse again!

"It's called an incidental finding."

"What is?" Now I'm starting to become more than irritated. Albert uses a freaking pen every single morning to make his list of what he needs to get done that day. Where the hell does he put the pen when he's done? Does he freaking eat it? Now I'm messing up a number of piles of mail, paperwork from the relocation, the rental agreement paperwork for the cottage and everything and anything that we have sort of neatly piled across the top of the kitchen table.

Suddenly Brad is done with all of the pausing and throat clearing and he just blurts out an entire paragraph. "The thing that showed up on the edge of the viewing area of your scan. There's something there. And we don't know what it is. But it's something that you need to get checked and evaluated. And of course it is probably benign. But you need to get it checked."

Did he just use the word benign?

Screw the pen!

What the hell did he just say?

"What? What do you mean? What is it?" Now he's got my attention. I swear to God he just said the word benign. I thought I heard him say it. Did I just imagine that?

"We don't know."

"Well what do you think? What could it be?" Why did he use that word? People only use the word benign when they're talking about a tumor, right? What the hell did he use that word for?

"It's beyond the scope of what we are familiar with here at the Orthopedic Center. It's something that the Radiologist noticed and he has recommended that you have follow up on it. You are going to want to contact your primary care doctor, explain to him that you have an incidental finding from an MRI of your right shoulder and you will need an x-ray of your chest."

"I don't have a primary care doctor." I just moved here. I have nothing. I don't even technically have my own address. I'm sort of homeless and alone in this state. Even though I'm still excited about being here. I just got here.

"Get one." His voice just got deeper.

"Okay." Now I'm the one pausing. I don't know what to say.

Brad's not talking.

"Thank you." It's all I can think of. I have no thoughts. And without thoughts I have no words. I swear to God I'm frozen. A huge wind of air from the Arctic Circle just blew through the tiny off-season rental cottage and it completely froze me solid. I can't move.

"Take care." Brad waited for me to say good-bye. He waited for like an entire minute because it's the polite thing to do. He must have thought the call dropped or something before he finally hung up the telephone.

I didn't say good-bye. And after I heard the click of Brad hanging up the telephone, I just quietly hung up. I don't remember ever doing that before.

Chapter 2

This cottage sucks!

I mean it's a place to live and all. It has everything we need. But it's not my home. And none of my stuff is here. I only have a suitcase full of clothes. That's all I brought when I moved here. I have none of my stuff! So every time I go to even make something for dinner, I find myself rummaging through the pan cupboard looking for the correct tools that I need for the creation. And none of the tools, which include the pans, pots, baking dishes and utensils are exactly what I'm looking for. They're not the things that I'm used to. I make do with them. But I'm growing tired of having to do that. I need to find a house and get the hell out of this cottage which is absolutely fine and wonderful and it's a place to live and I'm thankful to have it. I need to get back to my comfort zone which includes me being surrounded with all of my own stuff!

"What did they say?" Albert walked through the front door at the tail end of my conversation with the Orthopedic Center.

"The rotator cuff isn't torn!" I'm smiling as I dig through the cupboard in search of a freaking sauce pan so I can just make a simple can of soup!

"Oh?"

"That's the thing I was most concerned about." I stopped searching for the sauce pan for a split second and smiled at my husband. Albert's best friend recently tore his rotator cuff and had to have surgery followed by a whopping nine months of physical therapy. The entire process was way less than fun and exactly what I did not want Brad to tell me that I had.

"That's good then!" Albert's shuffling through the mess of paperwork that is scattered across the top of the table.

"Yeah he said there's some tendinitis and some sort of calcifications that are causing the pain." Where the hell is that sauce pan? I quickly return to my digging in the pan cupboard. The clanking and clanging is getting louder and louder. Why do I get the feeling that Albert's not even listening to me right about now. He's spotted the horrific mess of paperwork that I freaked over and spread across the table and most assuredly the clanging and clanking that I'm causing as I continue to dig for a sauce pan is just fueling his frustration. He's obsessing now and he's shuffling and sorting and shaking his head back and forth. He looks like he's looking for something. I'm hoping that is all it is. I'm nervous though. But realistically if he'd just left the freaking pen on the table after he finished using it so somebody else could maybe find it when they needed to use it none of this would have even happened! It's totally his fault. I'm just going to blame him if he mentions the mess. Funny thing is that I didn't even end up needing the stupid pen.

We used to have a cat that loved to mess up the piles of paperwork. And that cat was huge! I had brought him home when we moved into a two-hundred year old farmhouse, right here in New Hampshire, nearly twenty years ago and the first time I'd been relocated here. And I loved that house! So much character, great woodwork, wide planks for the floor, a small working kitchen off a huge dining room! But it had mice. Lots and lots of mice that rummaged their way through the teeny openings in the dirt-rock basement, up through the holes around the plumbing, through the cabinet doors that wouldn't stay completely shut and into my kitchen! So I had to get a cat. And this cat loved those mice! We had that cat for nearly ten years, until he became so sick that we had to have the poor thing put down. He'd probably caught a freaking disease from eating all of those mice!

"Good. So you're fine." Albert's still sorting through the mess. "Where the hell did I put that listing for the house off King Street?"

Are you freaking kidding me?! What the hell did Albert do with the one freaking sauce pan that this freaking cottage comes with? How can something completely disappear?! "Don't know."

"You don't know if you're fine?"

"I don't know where the listing for King Street is." Forget it! I just won't eat! I angrily slam the cupboard.

"How is it that when I put something on the table so I can find it later it can just up and disappear?! This whole table is a freaking mess!" Now Albert's angry.

Dammit! If I still had that freaking cat I would have an answer!

Chapter 3

I feel like I've been here forever. But I really just got here.

The streets are somewhat familiar and as I'm driving around looking for a place to live, every now and then I feel like I know where I am. Sort of like a feeling of "Deja Vu". In other words it's not just that I think I've driven down the road once before and more than likely twenty years ago when I lived in this area I did do just that; beyond that it's more like a feeling of discovery even though it's already familiar and perhaps somewhat expected.

It's like that feeling you get when you're sitting in your dark living room watching a horror movie. All of the lights are off and you're reaching the very end of the movie when all of the sudden the hair on the back of your neck stands up because you suddenly just know what horrific 'thing' is about to happen! Or it's like you're one person in a crowd of hundreds and you're each gripping hold of a ticket stub as a man with a microphone announces a series of nine numbers from the short edge of the winning raffle ticket. And by the time he reaches the sixth number you feel the same hairs on the back of your neck suddenly standing at attention because you for some reason just know that you are about to win!

At least that's the way it feels for me. It's a tingling sort of feeling that something is about to happen and for some reason you know what that thing is depending on the situation that you're in. And that thing that's about to happen can be a good thing or a bad thing. Either way you'll have already recognized it when it arrives. Either way the hair on the back of your neck will stand up. It's a fork in the road really. If you go to the right it will be bad but oh so familiar and recognizable. If you go to the left it will be good and again it will be familiar and recognizable. The outcome is not really the point. The feeling that you know something is about to happen is the point.

"Let's start with the properties in Laconia." Albert is steering and twisting the giant big man car along the bumpy dirt road that we temporarily live on.

"Want to start with King Street?" I'm tapping the GPS.

"No. I drove by this house yesterday and want to take a look at it."

"Oh. Okay." I've pretty much given up looking for a place to live. I actually arrived in New Hampshire a couple of months ago; before the family. Within the first week of getting here I'd already looked at dozens of houses and actually placed an offer on a property. It fell through when we got to the inspections. I was living in a hotel room offered by the company that transferred me here. They told me I could stay in the hotel as long as I needed to. That's another story altogether! Needless to say I'm in a short term rental as Albert and I continue to search for a place to live. Our house in Massachusetts sold. We're quite literally homeless even though we're renting. When you've owned a home for nearly thirty years and you suddenly find yourself living out of a suitcase with your husband, one of your five children (three, when the two that are in college come home) and the dog it feels like you're homeless. Maybe 'homeless' isn't the correct word; perhaps it's more a feeling of detachment. I guess I feel detached. Like I'm just floating around in the breeze. I'm getting nervous. I'm worried that if I don't find something quickly, the owner of the short term rental is going to tell me to get the hell out because the 'weekly rental season' will have arrived. At that point our only option will be to sleep in the two freaking vehicles we have with all of our clothes, a little bit of food and the dog. The 'weekly rental season' will be here very soon. The snow has nearly melted even though we are still battling with occasional and annoying snowstorms. But it's nearly done. It's almost Spring/Summer time when the tourists will invade the beautiful lakes of New Hampshire. And even after we find a home we will need to get under contract, get through inspections, schedule a closing, and get our stuff out of storage that is an entire state away from where we now are. All of that takes time, which we are running out of! We need to find a home!

"Where is this house?"

"It's actually very close to downtown. You can walk to it from downtown!" Albert's smiling. I'm not. I'm more of a 'hide me in the woods so I don't have to deal with any people' sort of person. I grew up in Maine for Christ's sake. I need woods and seclusion and peace and quiet. I need to be back in the day when the doorbell rang more than the telephone because the only way for people to connect with you was to pull into the driveway and wave at you as you pulled weeds from the garden out back. That was when the phones were attached to the wall, not to our hips.

"So what's the downtown like?" I'm trying to be a team player here.

"I'll drive you through it before we go to the house; it's actually right here." He spins the wheel around.

And boy was Albert right. With one twist of the wheel we suddenly found ourselves driving slow and steady through quaint brick buildings and sidewalks. A host of privately owned small businesses line the streets of downtown Laconia. And it's pretty! There's a deli, antique shops, boutiques, a barber shop, shops full of craft things, and second-hand stores! Just anything and everything you can imagine. I immediately picture myself strolling through the area with a cup of coffee and Violet on the end of her pretty purple puppy leash. This area could probably work!

"The house is at the end of this street." Just as we round the end of a rotary shaped downtown full of side streets, businesses and people that are nice we are already there and Albert pulls into a short driveway.

"This is it?"

"This is it." Albert jumps out of the car.

"It's on the water?!" My focus immediately leaps to the blue river running directly across the back of the property.

"That's my favorite part!" Albert is grinning ear to ear as we stumble over a small remaining snow bank and walk across the back yard. He and my second oldest son, who still lives with us, are both avid fishermen.

"Where does the river lead to?"

"Lake Winnisquam." More smiling on Albert's part. "And it is right over there." He points to the right and I can see that the river is swelling into the mouth of the lake just around a small bend in the waterway. Winnisquam is a completely gorgeous, deep and large lake! Having direct access to that is a huge victory if this house happens to work out.

"Wow!" Now I'm smiling.

"Let's check it out." Albert marches toward the front door just as a white SUV pulls into the driveway and the young man driving it wildly waves at him.

"How the hell is it that I'm missing all these details? You already set up the appointment?" I quickly follow Albert.

"Yep. I peeked in the windows yesterday. Gave the guy a call to get us into it."

"Great!" So far this is working out perfectly. And the minute we stepped inside it was obvious that the search was over. More than two thousand square feet, three floors, five bedrooms, four bathrooms and all it needs is paint, carpet and a good and thorough cleaning!

"Let's get the offer written up." Albert's speaking with the broker. "All cash. Close in two weeks."

"You got it!" The broker pulls out of the driveway and just like that we were on the way to salvation.

"What's the price again?"

"Eighty."

I shake my head in disbelief. "This is too good to be true!" How can it be that I've looked for two maybe three solid months straight for a place to call home and Albert strolls into town and immediately finds the perfect solution? Is he that much better at house shopping than me? Does he have a sixth sense for it? Whatever! Let's hope this one's a slam dunk! I'm grinning from ear to ear as I hop into the giant big man car with Albert.

"Yeah. This one will work just fine."

"How can the price be so low?" I'm still not believing it.

"Foreclosure." Albert's still smiling. I don't think he's stopped smiling since we pulled into the driveway.

"Perfect." I quietly leaned my head back onto the rest and sighed. Please let this one work out okay! We need to get comfortable. We need to have a home again. And as we pulled out of the driveway and back down the tiny road to downtown Laconia I had the most amazing feeling that somebody was watching over and guiding us. For some reason this home, at this time, in this town and in the State of New Hampshire is supposed to become our new home. The tiny little hairs on the back of my neck are standing up and I feel like something is about to happen.

Chapter 4

"The people at the Orthopedic Center say I need to find a primary care doctor." I'm sitting on the loveseat and staring across the living room at Albert when I bring up the subject. The subject that I was truly just planning on ignoring. The subject which in my mind would amount to nothing more than complete aggravation. And the aggravation would be based on the fact that once again the medical community had convinced me that I needed to pay for more and more tests, appointments and lab work which would ultimately become nothing more than the all too familiar statements involving my age and what's common amongst 'us' people. And then I would become even angrier with the entire escapade on the day when I finally would break down and write the check for probably thousands of dollars, which I would then send to the freaking medical office as thanks for telling me nothing more than, 'You're old.' And it dawned on me as I thought about the suggestions from Brad, that if he in fact had not used that one little word that he did I would have completely ignored him. That one word that caused me to say 'what did he just say' is truly the only reason I have decided to take his advice and get it double checked.

"Why?" He's watching television and holding the remote out in front of himself. His mouth is hanging open and his eyes are fixated. He has one foot propped up on the crazy looking coffee table, which I'm positive the owner of the cabin made herself. It's made of a half-piece of log and has three short stubby sticks on each end of it that protrude from the underside like a cactus of some sort. The thing is just ugly. Probably the majority of the people living within the woods of New Hampshire would see it as being a fabulous piece of country-junkified chic-ness.

"Because per usual doctor's offices just want me to waste all of my time and money for no reason whatsoever!" I sound angry. I feel confident that I'm correct, however.

Albert's still staring at the television. "Well what did they say?"

"They said there's a thing that showed up at the edge of the screen. They don't know what it is. They said I need to find a primary care doctor and have it followed up on. They said to get an x-ray of my chest." I'm literally rolling my eyes and snapping at Albert like it's his fault. I'm repeating a story that it feels like I've already read to him and he just wasn't paying attention. And of course this is complete ridiculousness on my part and Albert is innocently just trying to watch the television while he is now being forced to wonder what vicious beast has just crawled up my ass.

Albert's having a moment of silence now as he stares straight ahead and continues to grip hold of the remote, as if it's his lifeline. The remote is like his IV bag. Without it his body will shrivel and die because the IV bag is the deliverer of the nutrients and pain killers that he simply cannot exist without. The news has just come on. It's one of the only channels that we seem to get at this cottage. Actually there's like ten channels. I didn't even realize there were cable television packages out there that only include ten channels! I don't remember ever having only ten channels. Except when I was little and cable television didn't exist yet. In fact the television in this cottage almost looks exactly like the television my parents had bought when I was a little girl. Back then we had three channels but only two of them came in. Thankfully one of them was channel eight, which showed Disney movies on Sunday evenings. Of the ten channels that we have at this little off-season rental cabin, nine of them show programs that I didn't even think were still being shown. A couple of evenings ago I actually watched one of the episodes of 'Fantasy Island!' I was oddly thrilled! I felt like I slipped through a time portal and I was living my life from forty years ago but I'm now an adult; I'm no longer ten years old. Maybe that's why I like New Hampshire actually. It must have some sort of comforting feeling like coming home again even though it's not truly where I grew up. But it's close.

"What did they say?" He's stopped staring at the television. It's like the words I spoke have taken a good ten minutes to bore a hole through his skull and seep into his brain far enough that he finally recognized that the incessant buzzing around his head was in fact his wife talking and not an annoying mosquito.

"He used the word benign." I'm staring at the television

now. I'm done talking. Let's see what he does with that little tidbit of a detail.

"Who did?" I can see him staring at me, not the television, out of the corner of my eye. I'm not answering though. I'm trying to hear the news now.

"Who did you talk to?" More questions from Albert. I'm crossing my brow as I continue to stare at the television. I'm not interested in discussion and I'm positive that I'm being completely and horribly passively aggressive. I'm not as good as Albert is at this though. Quietly and nonchalantly Albert clicks the off button on the remote and places it onto the ugly but fabulously country-junkified chic coffee table.

"Brad."

"You talked to Brad?!" He's excited now. Albert is quite literally bouncing up and down in his chair. "When did Brad call?!"

Oh my God, I'm actually staring at Albert and fantasizing about flying across the tiny living room, snatching the remote from the coffee table while I'm in mid-air, and beating the top of his head to a pulp with it! "He's the one that called from the Orthopedic Center! Would you like me to tell him that you say 'HI' next time I talk to him? Actually, maybe the next time I talk to him I'll see if he would be willing to call you in a prescription of Ritalin."

Fortunately Albert chuckled before calmly asking me to explain what his 'I-wish-he-were-my-BFF' said.

"I'm sure it's nothing. But I should probably just get it checked. Just in case." I'm smirking when we both started to watch the news on the small and ineffective television in the off-season rental cottage that we call home in a State that for some reason feels like it is.

Chapter 5

"Do you want to go for a ride?"

Albert's just strolled out from the bedroom. I'm on my fourth cup of coffee and I've already taken Violet outside to do her business two times. The one of our five children that is still living with us full-time is fast asleep and I half expect will remain that way for at least three more hours.

"Where?" His mouth is huge as he yawns the question. How can he even open it that far? He looks like a hippo right now; I know it's mean of me to think that but that truly is what he looks like. It's either that or a PEZ dispenser. But the dispenser is tiny, fragile and brightly colored so as to attract toddlers that are standing in the checkout line with their mothers. Yeah, no. I'm calling it like it looks. He's a hippo.

"I want to check out a medical group in Laconia. I figured if it looks decent enough, I'll just go inside and fill out whatever paperwork I need to fill out to become a patient. Then I'll see about scheduling a follow up appointment for a chest x-ray." I can't see Albert anymore. He's in the kitchen and I can hear another yawn as he pours a cup of coffee. Why the hell is he so tired all of the time anyway? I think it's because of the snoring. His snoring is completely out of control. And it's really always been a 'thing' that I've just accepted over the years. I've actually gotten used to it. I remember years ago we had some house guests that were sleeping on the first floor of our house. Albert's and my bedroom was on the third floor of that particular house. When we all woke up the next day, I happily skipped down over the flights of stairs to make a delicious breakfast for our guests. I was smiling when I asked them if they had slept well and I was frowning when they answered the question.

"What is wrong with Albert?!" They were both staring at me as one of them responded.

"Huh?" I was so completely and utterly confused. The expressions across their faces were of anger. They looked as if they hadn't slept in a week. Their mouths were hanging open and their heads were leaning so far forward as they glanced up at me, that I thought they'd lost control of the muscles in their necks.

"That snoring!!!" One of them was almost yelling.

"How can you stand it!!!?" That other one was definitely yelling.

"What are you talking about?" I laughed as I answered them and I actually thought for a moment that perhaps they were just joking.

After years of listening to Albert's snoring become worse and worse as he's aged, I now find myself sneaking videos of him doing it, kicking the side of the bed to see if he will just stop, and on occasion just sitting up in bed and completely staring at him and wondering how any person in the world can possibly be getting any real sleep as the oxygen just continues to be depriving his brain of the nutrients it needs. It's no wonder he's always so freaking tired! It's no wonder he stares at the television for ten minutes before he actually hears my questions or statements. The fact that he snores instead of sleeping really amounts to nothing more than his body struggling to keep itself alive while at the same time it does nothing more than continue to try and kill him!

He needs to get that checked!

"Sure." He's walking into the living room with the giant big hippo mouth again. "Just let me wake up some."

I'm snickering as I skip through the living room, into the bedroom and ultimately into the master bathroom. "I'm taking a shower. We'll leave in thirty minutes!"

Chapter 6

The hippo mouth is driving the big man car down the road as we pull into the quaint little town of Laconia. And the moment I think about the description of my poor husband I scold myself within my own mind about continuing to look at him that way when he yawns. 'I have to stop this!'

"It should be on the other side of the rotary, on that road that leads toward Gilford, I think." I'm trying to remember what the map showed when I searched for a local medical group on line. "I think it should be a decent size building. It looked like there are surgeons, internists, foot doctors, and everything there. I'm hoping it is one of those places that if you go in and need lab work or an x-ray that they just do it all right there. Sort of one stop medical needs shopping!" I'm smiling as I turn toward my husband and once again see nothing but the hippo mouth. Dammit!

"What's it called?" He's leaning forward and he's trying to find the place as he continues to struggle with his fatigue.

"Why are you so tired?" He's starting to annoy me. "Oh, there it is!" Quickly I spot the facility and we immediately turn into the parking lot. The parking is completely crazy and confusing. Not so much from traffic but from design. We drove around the entire thing at least three times before we actually figured out where the entrance to the building was and therefore which row and direction it would make sense to park in.

"I like it. It's smaller than a hospital." I'm smiling as we begin to walk toward the entranceway.

"I think it's that bed." Albert's giant hippo yawn is screaming across the parking lot.

"What?"

"I'm not sleeping because of that freaking bed!"

"Yeah. It is as hard as a rock!" I'm laughing as we approach a reception desk for the entire building. I'm laughing not at the fact that the bed is horrible, which it truly is completely just that; I'm laughing at the fact that it has taken Albert at least ten minutes to even answer the question that I really didn't even think registered within his groggy mind. But the truth of the matter is that even if the bed were the best of all beds Albert would still be tired. It's the snoring. I'm sure of it.

"Good morning." The two ladies behind the desk are so pleasant and both smile.

"Hello there." Albert and I are both immediately comfortable. We like people that are nice. That's about all it takes for us to settle into a new place. "We're not sure where to go but we came by this morning because we are new to the area and we need to find a primary care doctor."

The two lovely ladies gave us instruction on where to go to fill out new patient paperwork and how to go about choosing a primary care physician from the list of available doctors. And literally within thirty minutes we had filled everything out, found a new doctor and had an appointment scheduled for me to be back tomorrow to be examined and hopefully have a chest x-ray! And the even better news is that the house we have put the offer on is right around the corner from the medical center.

"Do you want to go get some lunch somewhere?" As we maneuver through the parking lot, I'm feeling like we have a light at the end of our relocation tunnel. Things are feeling like they're starting to come together. Not like when we relocated to Massachusetts. We just aren't the type of people that become comfortable living in an area that's full of drugs, crime, and lots and lots of noise. I never really felt like I was home when we lived there. Even though I've technically only been in the State of New Hampshire for about four months so far and I'm still living out of a suitcase because I have no house to call my own but somehow I'm already feeling like I'm home.

"Let's stop by the real estate office and see if they've heard anything back on the offer." Albert's always thinking and quickly pulls the giant big man vehicle out of the parking lot. Just across town is the real estate office and it dawns on me that once we move into this little town we really won't need to go anywhere else. Everything is centrally located and the town itself is tiny enough that we can quite literally walk to wherever we need to go. Not that we will but we can if we so choose.

Literally like two minutes later we were walking into the real estate office. I'm loving the smallness of this pretty town and am chomping at the bit to know if our offer has been accepted or not!

"Hello. Is Frank available?" I'm smiling as I approach the receptionist and for some reason find myself immediately wondering what exactly her title is. Maybe she is an Executive Assistant? Or maybe she's an Administrative Assistant? Maybe she's the Office Manager? It's funny how titles change after years of a title being just fine with no complaints whatsoever. Why the change? Was it actually insulting for a person to be called a stewardess, or a receptionist, or a cashier for that matter? And now if a person that's older than fifty accidentally calls a person by the original title, he or she has unwittingly slammed that person right across the face with a slapping insult thereby ruining the 'receptionists' entire day or week or even month! I'm sure if I were to call the lady behind the desk in front of me right now a receptionist she would immediately become angry and insulted from my pure ignorance and in all likelihood would not even check to see if Frank is available or not. She'd tell us that he's in a meeting and that she'll be sure to get a message to him. Which of course she wouldn't! She'd jot a scribble of something down onto a sticky note and she'd angrily crumple it and toss it into the garbage can immediately upon our exit of the front office.

"Let me just see. And who can I say is asking for him?" There's a huge smile across her face and unfortunately she has a massive smear of thick red lipstick coating her teeth as well as her lips. The coffee cup in front of her has rancid and obviously cold coffee from the start of her morning and the lipstick on the cup is even thicker than what remains on her lips and teeth.

Politely I explain who we are as Albert starts humming and strolling through the office. The 'receptionist' quickly scoots from behind her desk and heads down a short hallway towards a handful of tiny offices. As I turn to look at Albert I find myself becoming completely annoyed with the fact that per usual he is bobbing his head up and down as he is humming. And the most annoying part of the entire scene is the fact that there is no music playing.

"Hey, how's it going?" Frank is standing in the reception area smiling and invites Albert and me to follow him down the tiny hall.

As quickly as we entered Frank's office, he turned to us and exclaimed that the bank had in fact accepted our offer. My bottom hadn't even touched the chair and I found myself immediately standing back up, thanking Frank, and skipping back down the tiny hallway to the open office space, where we told the 'receptionist' to have a good day before we left.

I can see the light at the end of the tunnel and its rays seem to be embracing me with a comforting hug. Things are going to be okay.

Chapter 7

After getting the great news about our soon to be home last evening, Albert and I had gotten a quick dinner at one of the local restaurants. We felt compelled to celebrate! After dinner we drove over to our new house and parked the giant big man car across the street while we stared at it. We watched as a handful of people walked by and probably ninety-percent of them turned a sharp left after passing our house and walked along the railroad tracks and over a rickety bridge that leads to a neighborhood across the river. And the nice thing is that our house isn't really in a neighborhood. It feels like it's in a secluded area even though it's not secluded at all because it is what one would call a 'downtown house'. And the other neat thing is that it sits directly on the road. Literally the front lawn is a sidewalk. But even though it sits directly on the road, you cannot see a thing in the back yard. There's a rod-iron fence and a thick bushel of tall trees that surround the edge of backyard that runs along the sidewalk. And along the side of the property is an even thicker group of trees creating a tall wall that separates the back yard from the train tracks, which I don't believe have been used for a great number of years. The property is protected even though it is completely exposed. I find this such an interesting balance that as we sit and continue to stare at our home I fall head over heels in love with it. I can't wait to move in. This is exactly where we are supposed to be. The house is perfect!

And now this morning Albert and I are driving by our protected and perfect new home before rounding the corner by the police station, taking one tiny left hand turn and suddenly finding ourselves parking the giant big man car in the crazy and confusing parking lot at the medical center.

"They need to redesign this freaking parking lot." I'm chuckling as Albert somehow manages to find a parking spot directly across from the entrance. How does he do that? I never find good parking spots. And it's because I know that about myself that I instinctually park in the very first spot I see because I know it is a fruitless mission to drive in monotonous circles, waiting and hoping for a better position that will do nothing but save me from walking an additional twenty feet. What's the point? It's only twenty feet! But Albert manages to hit the parking spot lotto every single time we go anywhere. And every single time he does I find myself so thankful that he saved us the additional twenty feet. This is probably why for almost thirty years I've just accepted that he's always the one to drive. It's not because he drives better than me because I honestly think I am truly the better driver. I don't speed at all. I'm extremely conscientious and considerate of other drivers. Albert has had way more car accidents than I have so clearly I am the better driver yet we both have come to accept without question that he will drive the giant big man car when we go someplace together. It's really all about the parking spots!

The same lovely ladies from yesterday greet us as we enter the medical center. They explain to us how to get to our new doctor's office and we very quickly find ourselves sitting comfortably in a pretty blue and orange waiting room. There are at least ten other people waiting to see either doctors or nurses and there's a television playing the morning news that everybody seems to be staring at. Which is perfect for Albert and I because that means they won't notice us staring at them. Almost the second we sat and I began to develop my opinions from observation of the strangers in the waiting room, a nurse suddenly appeared at the doorway to the hidden offices and called my name.

"Holy smokes that was fast," I chuckled as Albert and I both stood and quickly followed the nurse through the door.

"How are you today?" The nurse is smiling and literally bouncing her way around the second waiting room that Albert and I are sitting in. She directs me to the examination table and begins to take my vital signs.

"I'm good thanks." I like her.

"What brings you in today?"

"Well, I am new to the area."

"Oh WOW. Where are you from?" She sounds surprised that anybody would move to the area, which I immediately don't understand. This is one of the most beautiful areas that I have ever seen, except for Hawaii. How on earth is she surprised that we are here? There are views from every street of the most beautiful mountains. There are woods and lakes everywhere. This area is so breath-taking and even though I've only been back in New Hampshire for just a few short months, I've already seen some of the most breathtaking sunsets of my life. How can she not see the beauty that is quite literally screaming all around her?

"We moved here from Massachusetts but I'm actually from Maine." I would never tell anybody that I was from Massachusetts. And the question 'where are you from?' feels like the person is asking where you have originated from. But it also feels like they want to know where you just were. So I always answer the question in two ways and at the same time I remain quite pleased and comfortable announcing to people that I'm a true 'Mainer'. That is something to brag about as far as I'm concerned. People from Maine live life the way it ought to be! Or at least we're supposed to. I've got a little bit of work to do on this one, obviously. But I'm still going to brag about it. I'm in the club. And you can't be in that club unless you were born and raised in the state. There aren't that many of us. And that's a good thing!

"What part of Maine?" She's still smiling and her body is forever quivering as she continues to bounce up and down. It's like the bouncing gives her life. She just can't stop because if she stops she will in all likelihood stop breathing. She must have been a cheerleader at some point in her life and it must have been a highlight for her because she can't quite shake it off.

"Well, I was born in Calais which is on the border to Canada. But when Albert and I lived there we were in the mid-coast area."

"What part of the mid-coast area?" She's still bouncing as she takes my blood pressure.

"The Brunswick area."

"Where's that?"

"About an hour north of Portland." This conversation is never going to end and I'm actually beginning to become annoyed with her. I'm going to have to take control. "So about a month or so ago I began having trouble with my shoulder and recently went to an Orthopedic Center for it; they did an MRI."

"Okay." The bouncing has suddenly stopped. It's like a light switch just got turned off and she's standing completely solid as she studies my face with her piercing eyes. Her mouth is no longer smiling and she's clamped her lips shut as her cheek muscles tighten around her face. That light switch clearly controlled the 'on or off' for the bouncing cheerleader and now the nurse is here!

I calmly told my story and smiled when I got to the part about receiving instructions from Brad to find a primary-care physician and get an x-ray of my chest.

"Oh, wow! Okay." She's begun to quickly type on a little laptop computer that's sitting on the counter top in the examination room.

"And here we are." Now I'm bouncing and smiling as I swing my legs to and fro while they dangle off the edge of the table that I'm sitting on.

"The doctor will be right in." And just like that she was gone. The nurse and her fluffy frantic pompoms have left the room.

"Chatty Cathy." I'm chuckling as I look at Albert who surprisingly hasn't said a single word. "I wonder if she comes with extra dresses and a tiny set of dishes." No response whatsoever from Albert. What the hell is wrong with him? He's supposed to be talking so I don't have to. He's just sitting there and he's looking around the room. He's not even humming, even though there's music playing! Why isn't he humming?

"How are you today? I'm Doctor Woods." Suddenly he's there. I've got to give this office a lot of credit for their efficiencies. I've literally been here for no more than fifteen minutes and I'm already seeing the doctor.

"Hello. Nice to meet you." I like him already. He just has that look that tells me he's wicked smart and that smile that tells me he's wicked nice.

"What brings you in today?"

Here we go again. I calmly and correctly repeat the same story that I just shared with the nurse and I finished the story by telling the doctor that the Orthopedic Center had recommended I find a primary care doctor and get an x-ray of my chest. As I wrapped up the final few words of that statement, however, is probably when I accidentally pissed off my new doctor.

"Well the great thing about this particular medical facility is that we treat the patient not the story." He's smiling as he spins around and washes his hands in the tiny little sink that sits in the very corner of the examination room.

"Okay." Oh great. I made him mad. For some reason doctors don't like to feel as if somebody else is telling them how to do their job. I'm not so sure I like him anymore. But I need something from him so I decide to just continue and present my polite self as if I'm on stage. I feel like I'm back at work, at the front of the store and I just came upon a pissed off customer. Now I need to rectify the situation! But this time I'm the one that caused the situation to actually happen!

"Let's examine the patient now and see where that gets us." He's still smiling.

Within less than three minutes the examination was over and amounted to a quick listen of my lungs and a few movements of my aching shoulder and about a dozen questions or statements, to which I responded with a smile, nod and a polite ass kissing statement such as, "Oh, really? I didn't know that!" Through the entire examination the doctor was still smiling. He actually has a beautiful smile! He explained that the facility can do the x-ray right down the hall and then he would meet us in his office and we would look at the x-ray together.

"Great!" I quickly hopped up and off the examination table and skipped my way down the hall toward the radiology department. Albert quietly followed along and waited in a small hallway waiting spot as the x-ray was completed. And when I say it's a 'waiting spot' that is literally all it is. There are two chairs that have been placed along the wall in the hallway just outside the door to the giant x-ray machine. I remember the days of getting x-rays and every scrap of metal needed to be removed from our bodies. Sort of like cooking food in a microwave. The metal stuff just wasn't allowed in there. Everything came off: ear-rings, rings, belts, bras with an under wire. But on this particular day I literally walked in fully clothed and "blinged-out" to the x-ray screen, stood perfectly still, took in a big breath, and boom! The picture was complete.

"Now just go back the way you came and enter the first office on your left. Doctor Woods will meet you there." The lady taking the x-ray held her arm out as she directed me toward the door and out of her x-ray room. I know she has a title that has something to do with radiology but I can't for the life of me remember what it is.

Albert is quietly sitting there waiting for me.

"What do you call the people that take the x-ray?" It's just a curiosity and it's under my skin now.

"What?" I think I just woke Albert up.

"What do they call those people?"

"What people?" He's almost stumbling as he stands up out of the chair. Was he just freaking sleeping? I think I see some drool on the front of his shirt. My God I was only in there for like two minutes. How could he have taken a nap?

"Never mind." Some things just aren't even worth explaining. By the time you finish trying to figure out what you were asking about and you actually explain it well enough to the person you are soliciting for help with the query, the amount of energy expelled in doing so just wasn't worth losing and for that matter you are just no longer interested in figuring it out.

It dawns on me that perhaps the reason for the stumbling on Albert's part is because of his right knee. About six months ago it had suddenly swelled up to the size of a freaking football just lying across the front of his leg. And then all of the sudden I was promoted, we were moving, and he had to pack the entire house by himself. He had gone to the doctor and was told that there is an injury; something about a meniscus. But that's where it stopped. Who has time to deal with injuries when life is so incredibly busy? Not Albert. Not me.

"Is this the right office?" Albert and I made our way to the doctor's office and it feels weird that we are meeting him in this environment. Why not back to an examination room? Maybe this is the only computer that will be able to show us the x-ray? Maybe the laptop in the examination room doesn't have the right program on it?

"How we doing?" The doctor is back and promptly sits behind his desk. Immediately he pulls up the x-ray and twists the computer screen slightly towards Albert and me as we sit in creaky wooden chairs across the desk from him. "Okay, here we show your rib cage."

"Okay." I'm sitting on the edge of my seat but not in the literal sense. I'm ready to hear that we have completely wasted our time. There's never anything wrong with me when doctors send me in for 'just in case' tests. And I'm utterly convinced that the entire medical community is nothing but a great big group of scammers and they are all just trying to get more money from me. And it's not like my insurance won't cover it but my insurance along with the entire country's will continue to rise in price because of all the unnecessary testing that we continue to perform when it is completely not necessary whatsoever!

"We have an issue."

"Huh?" What the hell did he just say?

"Right here." He's pointing at something that to me looks like nothing but swirls of white, gray and black matter. I can tell there are ribs but that's all I see.

"What is it?"

"I don't know." He's looking at me. "You're going to need to have a C Scan."

"Why?" Now I'm literally standing up. Forget the edge of the seat. I want an explanation. What the hell is he looking at? What the hell is he talking about? What the hell is the issue?

"Okay, see right here." His voice is calm as he continues to look at my eyes and he points directly to the computer screen.

"Yes."

"See how on this side of your chest the line on the edge is smooth and straight?"

"Yes." I'm walking to the other side of his desk.

"And see how on this other side of your chest that line looks all round. It sort of looks like the letter 'B'?" He's looking up at me as he points with a pen to the area he is describing.

"Yes." I'm literally standing over him as I've completely maneuvered myself around and to the backside of his desk.

"That's an issue."

"Well what kind of issue?" My hands are on my hips now and I feel like I'm scolding one of my children.

"I don't know." He's blinking as he looks up at me and continues to sit in his beautiful leather bound fancy doctor's office chair.

"What is it?"

"I don't know but we need to find out. It's not supposed to look like that."

"Well what could it be?" The front of my legs are literally

leaning against the arm of his chair and I'm just staring at the x-ray. Below me I see him out of the corner of my eye as he waves his hands in the air a bit and shakes his head back and forth. But I'm not focusing on him at all now. I'm just staring straight ahead at the computer screen and I'm glaring at the edge of my lung that is shaped like the letter 'B'.

"It could be anything."

"Well, like what?" Now I'm glaring at this poor man.

"It could be TB. It could be Mesothelioma."

"What?" I'm laughing now. Even the thought of TB is completely ridiculous to me. And as far as Mesothelioma goes; isn't that the thing I see TV commercials about? Isn't that the thing that people get if they worked in a freaking factory that made asbestos like a hundred years ago?

He's not laughing. His mouth is shut and he's looking up at me.

And now the room is quiet.

"Okay so where do we go for the C Scan." Mr. Silence has finally decided to speak and I almost forgot Albert was even in the room.

"We will set it up and call you. The C Scan will be read by one of the surgeons in our center and we'll schedule you for that appointment as well. You'll have the C Scan right at the hospital and then you'll come in and meet with the surgeon after that."

"Okay." Albert's the one speaking now and I have suddenly assumed the role of silence. And now that 'Mr. Used-to-be-Silent' is speaking I'm wondering why he isn't questioning this nimrod of a doctor about the fact that I have to go see a surgeon! Why does a surgeon have to be the one that I see after the C Scan? Why can't he be the one to read the scan results to me? Has he already made the assumption that I'm going to NEED a surgeon? That's not freaking happening! I haven't even finished moving yet! I just freaking got here!!

"While you're here we should do a TB test and we'll have you come back tomorrow for the injection site to be read by one of the nurses."

"Okay." Did I really just say 'okay'? What the hell is wrong with me? I'm getting completely pissed off and I'm not even sure why! A TB test is completely stupid! Another way to get more money from me or the insurance company! And that's all it is! Why do I have to freaking do that? And as all of these thoughts full of rage race through the neurons in my brain, I decide to take a deep breath and try and force my psyche to 'just relax already'! Slowly I move out from behind the doctor's desk. I've decided I should probably give the man some space and quietly moved back to my chair next to Albert.

"Okay so I'll have the nurse come right in and she'll administer the TB test. Good luck with everything." He's smiling again. I can feel his discomfort but I'm not sure if it's because he just gave me some concerning news or if he's uncomfortable with me. And then he was gone.

Albert and I sat in our chairs and waited for the nurse to come in and stick me with a needle. And it was so incredibly quiet in that office. We were just looking around the room. There was no humming and no head bobbing. And for some reason I had just at that moment begun to actually listen to the music playing throughout the medical center. It was pleasant and very soft. I wondered why I hadn't listened to the music until just at that moment. Maybe that was the only moment that my thoughts had actually quieted down, thereby giving me enough peace that I actually heard the music? I closed my eyes for like a nano-second and felt my head slowly beginning to bob up and down to the beat of the very pleasant music.

Then it hit me and I shook my head back and forth with vigor as I half expected that I would begin to hum the music! My thoughts were suddenly awake again. I could feel my brain slamming into the sides of my skull and I could feel my blood beginning to boil to the point that the edges of my throat burned with rage. There was no reason whatsoever for any of this! Why am I continuing to follow along with this complete charade? This is perhaps the most ridiculous situation I've ever been sucked into! I am going to completely freak on all of the medical people involved in this when it's all over and they tell me that there's nothing wrong.

I turned toward Albert who just sat in silence again. He was staring straight ahead and he offered no words at all. Whatever thoughts were racing, or in fact maybe they were just crawling, through his brain he was keeping to himself. And as I stared at him, I could feel the rage beginning to boil just beneath the surface of my very being!

"What a complete freaking waste of time!"

Chapter 8

I remember years ago when I brought my second child, who was only two years old at the time, in to the doctor for a "well-care" visit. The nurse measured his head, took his weight, height and vitals. When the doctor came in and read the results he immediately expressed concern over my son's head measurement. He said that the measurements were not following the 'arc in the graph' like he would have expected. He said that he wanted to have a C Scan done of my son's head to make sure that the plates were not fusing prematurely. For the next three days, as I waited for that appointment, I sat and watched my son playing like any other normal child and I fought back the tears. I was a complete train wreck!

When we finally got to the appointment at the largest hospital in the entire state of Maine, I remember speaking with the Radiologist immediately after the test had been taken. He looked at me and he said, "Why are you here?"

Everything was fine. I was thankful for that of course and at the same time I was thankful that the Pediatrician was being more than thorough in double-checking that my child was okay. But what a three day period of time! As harsh as it sounds when I think about this incident I can't help but think what a horrible and torturous waste of time it all was. I thank God for the outcome, of course, but I can't shake the almost anger that I feel because the reality was that nothing was wrong and I spent days worrying and money that I didn't have to spend. Those three days were probably three of the hardest I've ever had. My world felt as if it would collapse if there was something wrong with one of my children. Those three days were truly my definition of what it is like to be completely terrified.

Oddly I do not feel that way about myself. Well for one it's not a three day waiting period. The doctor's office called about two hours after the x-ray of my chest to let me know that I was already scheduled at the hospital for the C Scan; I was scheduled for the very next day and here we are driving to that appointment. Unlike the feeling of terror that I felt when we were double-checking the plates of my son's skull, this time I just feel like I know there will be nothing wrong. I know that this is a complete waste of time and I can't stop feeling completely annoyed. I feel like I'm wasting my money. I feel like it's all a big scam to make me pay for huge expensive tests that are going to do nothing but show that there is nothing wrong with me. My shoulder hurts. That's it! And it's weird the way I'm more concerned with the money than myself. But for some reason that is what my mind is hanging its hat on. Those thoughts are fueling my rage for having to drive to another medical facility and spend another afternoon or morning of my time doing things that I really don't have to and don't want to. Why is that? Am I not worth the extra checking? I'm pretty sure I am worth it. But it doesn't feel like I should be focusing on myself just yet. Why are these my thoughts? I sort of feel like I know why I can't get my head around the possibility that anything could ever be wrong with me. I'm thinking that perhaps the reason is, that I just know within my heart and mind that I am not one of 'those people'. I never have been. I never will be. Nothing is ever going to happen to me. I'm one of the ones that reads about the others. I'm one of the ones that is never impacted by tragedy. I'm one of the ones that always survives. I sort of feel like I'm Superman; even though I'm a girl. And there's no such thing as kryptonite on the planet. And there's no danger that kryptonite is suddenly going to show up because there are no evil villains flying to earth from a far-away galaxy with a bag full of the element so they can attempt to take me down. I'm always going to be okay. I'm invulnerable. I'm not one of the others. I AM Superman. Therefore these appointments are stupid.

As Albert pulls the giant big man car into the parking lot at the hospital, I can't help but once again feel that the design of another parking lot is completely crazy! The hospital is actually a beautiful building with lots of big glass windows and doors across the front. It sits high on a hill and right in the middle of a residential neighborhood. And the sun is completely gorgeous today, which makes the building itself look even prettier than it probably usually does. It looks like a little cousin to the Emerald City for goodness sakes!

"This is pretty."

"Yep." Albert's still being unusually quiet. He normally

doesn't stop talking. Especially to strangers. We know this!? And I'm actually relieved that he isn't talking because I'm completely not in the mood to listen to him. And if he were talking I probably would just be nodding my head and saying 'mm-hmm' even though I would have no idea whatsoever what he would be talking about. And I'm positive it would have no special meaning to me whatsoever anyway! And as the giant big man car continues to circle the parking lot in search of an acceptable spot, I find myself suddenly becoming oddly irritated with the fact that once again Albert has managed to park in the most perfect spot. We are literally twenty feet from the entrance to the building of glass! How can he always find these perfect parking spaces and why for the love of God can I not?!

As we walk into the building we are greeted by a host of very nice people that direct us, take my medical and insurance information and make us feel wonderfully comfortable. Once again I am more than impressed with the efficiency of the entire process of showing up, registering and taking any sort of medical test. I literally sat in the waiting room for three minutes before being called in for my scheduled procedure. Every hospital in the country needs to take a lesson from the medical offices and professionals in this town! They consistently are nailing it as far as I'm concerned! And when the day comes and they finally tell me that everything is normal and okay, I will probably forgive them for wasting my time because I am so loving the management of their processes and their customer service right now! I won't forgive them for the poorly designed parking lots though. That one I'm just going to keep shaking my head about as I wonder what in tarnation the local planning board was thinking about when they approved the designs.

"Why are you here?" The girl guiding me through the hallways to the great big machine that I'm about to slide into is smiling and bouncing. I think everybody that enters the medical field in this town was a cheerleader when they came through either the Middle School or the High School.

"I had something unusual show up on an MRI and a chest x-ray." I'm chewing gum and trying not to slurp as I answer her questions.

"Everything from the waste up off, put on this Johnny and

then come back out."

I immediately realize that she was only asking me why I was here to make sure she was speaking with the correct patient. "Okay. What about jewelry?"

"What do you have?" She's still smiling.

"Rings."

"They're okay. Do you have a belt on?"

"No."

"You're all set then."

She closes the door and I follow her instructions before coming back out. How can it be that rings are okay but a belt wouldn't be? Is it the size of metal that matters? Is it the placement of metal because my hands will rest far enough away from where they'll be 'x-raying' but a belt buckle wouldn't? Per usual I'm confused. Isn't this machine like a giant magnet or something? Years ago when I had spinal surgery, they fused a couple of vertebrae together with a cadaver bone and a metal plate. What if the machine tries to suck the metal plate in my neck right through my flesh and I just die on the table? How come that metal is okay? Is it a different kind of metal from a belt buckle? When I filled out the paperwork, I remember listing it on the history part. Did anybody read that information? Why would they ask if it weren't important? Is this how it is going to all end for me? Has that ever happened to anybody? They laid down for the C Scan and within minutes their body imploded making the machine look like a freaking maniac had charged through the hospital doors, down the hall, into the radiology department, through the very doors that I just walked through, and in a rage of horrific psychedelic mania chopped up a body like a goddamn sausage with a freaking machete!

"What about the metal I have in my neck?" I can actually hear my voice quivering when I speak to the nurse. My Johnny is wrapped tightly around my body and I'm completely freezing when I walk into the room which is basically empty except for a giant donut-shaped machine with a sliding narrow table.

"That kind of metal is non-magnetic. You'll be fine. Are you cold?"

I just stared at her as I clocked my head to the right and thought to myself, 'Then why did you ask for that information when I filled out the paperwork?' I ignored my thoughts. I immediately focused on the logic behind her comment that 'that type of metal is non-magnetic.' What kind of metal is non-magnetic, anyway? This seems weird. I thought it all was magnetic. I remember when I was in fourth grade science class and we were testing things with a giant magnet. We pressed the magnet up against wood and nothing happened. We pressed the magnet up against a piece of paper and nothing happened. We pressed the magnet up against METAL and something happened! I don't remember anything about certain kinds of metal behaving differently when a magnet was pressed up against them! Was I just not paying attention? I don't remember failing science class as a child though! She's wrong! She's making a mistake!

The tiny smiling and forever bouncing nurse directs me to lie down on the table. She covered me with a long white blanket that felt as if it had just been pulled from a microwave oven. It was so incredibly warm and exactly what I needed as I tried to calm down and I figured that is exactly why the nurse placed it on me and I imagine that she does the same thing for every patient. Slowly, I begin to relax. I take a deep breath and just decide to try and nap while they slide me into and out of the great big spinning hole in the machine. I tell myself that everything is going to be okay and I remind myself that the professionals are taking care of me and they wouldn't ever let something happen to one of their patients, while they're simply sliding them into and out of the giant donut. My mind was calming down and I was no longer in a frozen state of panic. Quietly and monotonously I breathed. And as I breathed I tried to concentrate on the new house and how wonderful it will be when we have all of our belongings in place and I actually get to cook a delicious dinner for my family again. As I think and as I dream I can feel my body as it lies on the narrow sliding table, slowly being pulled or pushed back and forth as I am being slid into the giant donut. The movement completely distracted my thoughts away from the new house and without thinking I opened my eyes to verify what was happening. And the second I focused on the giant machine I unfortunately became completely and utterly immersed within the frozen state of panic yet again! The giant hole that my body slid through was spinning and humming over and around my head. As the machine spun around and around my thoughts raced in tandem with the movement. My thoughts ran as fast as they could possibly run around and around in a giant circle within my head. My thoughts seemed to be a jumble of panic and flailing arms but they truly were only one singular being that continually screamed and vibrated within the walls of my feeble brain. The screaming was intense and the screaming was loud and the screaming continually cried out to myself that I was truly about to die! The metal in my neck is going to be sucked through my flesh and I am going to die! I can feel the pressure! I can feel it like a pulsating thrust of pressure against the back side of my frail splintering spine! It's moving! The freaking metal plate in my neck is moving and it's going to explode with a burst of horrific spewing and spitting blood through the very surface of my soft satiny skin! This is it!

And then the music came on. And it was loud but it was quiet. It was just enough of a distraction that my mind jumped to the beat of the music as it piped through the speaker system. A soft country western song played throughout the room and began to soothe the very depths of my horrific paranoia! Suddenly I heard a different voice speaking directly to me: 'take a deep breath and hold it.' Silently I followed the words and did as I was told. And for the mere moments that I held my breath, I suddenly felt that I was calming down and everything was going to be okay. Is that the reason they tell patients to take a deep breath? Is it their way of forcing us to all just calm down for a minute? Is there no medical reason behind the instruction whatsoever except to relax the patient so they can get clear images? My neck was not exploding, the metal plate was fixed as it always has been against the vertebra within my neck, and my breathing remained calm and monotonous. Within twenty minutes it was over and I found myself wondering if I'd fallen asleep and my raging thoughts had been nothing more than a nightmare. Perhaps I'd slept through eighty percent of the test and now suddenly I was getting dressed to leave.

As I strolled back through the hallway and into the waiting area I immediately noticed that Albert was sprawled across his chair, had his legs outstretched, his shirt twisted up around his belly and his arms flopped out from his sides. There was a long puddle of drool soaking the front of his white and light blue checkered button-down shirt and his head rested toward his left shoulder.

"You ready to go?" I'm looking around the room to see how many people are smirking and chuckling at the sleeping Albert. I'm disappointed that the one little old lady that is sharing the room with him is only filling in the letters of a cross-word puzzle. She hasn't even noticed him; or perhaps she did but she really doesn't care. I of course, if I were her, would still be staring and would have made up an entire episode of a day in the life of Albert within my mind. I'm not sure what sort of story I would come up with about Albert though. Why would he be sleeping in the waiting room? He doesn't really look like a scary individual that perhaps would be hiding from the law and has just slithered in off the streets to sleep in the waiting room because of complete exhaustion from hiding and running all night. He doesn't really look like he's completely disheveled and wrinkled because he has been waiting for a loved one to get out of surgery for the last eight hours. He certainly doesn't look like he works in the hospital; he's not wearing scrubs. He looks too ordinary. He just looks like a guy that sat down and took a nap as he sat crookedly in a waiting room chair. And as I would continue to stare at him I would eventually come to reason that his sleeping is from pure laziness more than anything else. He's sleeping because he has nothing going on. He's sleeping because he is completely bored. He's not worried about my tests either. If he were he'd be sitting at attention, while one of his knees bounced up and down. That's it. It is official: Albert thinks I'm Superman, too!

"You all done?" He startles himself awake and wipes the drool away from his chin.

"Yep. All done."

And as I stared at him and watched him pull his heavy body from the crooked stance he held across the waiting room chair, I wondered for a split second if maybe I was wasting his time as much as the doctors that were ordering these tests were wasting mine. Why did I have to have him come with me?

Together we exited the pretty glass covered hospital, jumped into the giant big man car and drove across town so the nurse at my new doctor's office could look at the injection site on my arm from yesterday and tell me that I don't have TB.

Chapter 9

With all of the useless medical appointments wasting my time, you'd think I'd actually forgotten that I have a new job in a new store and am preparing to move into a new home. Timing is absolutely everything isn't it? Why does everything have to happen at the same time I wonder? These are the thoughts that roll through my brain as I twist the steering wheel of the Lincoln and enter the parking lot of the store that I work at now. Way off in the distance are the most beautiful mountains which frame the panoramic skyline of New Hampshire. It's completely breath-taking to look at every morning as I drive to work. The air is cool and crisp even though it's warm enough that the snow continues to melt. There are just a few cars from sales associates in the parking lot because we don't open for another thirty minutes. And it's quiet as I click my heels across the damp pavement. Tomorrow I go to meet a surgeon and find out that nothing substantial is on the C Scan, but today I need to focus on presenting myself to a group of people that know nothing about me.

It has been just a few short months of working with this new group of people. And for the most part they are completely wonderful. They are genuine, they have a passion for what they do, and they are committed to delivering results. I find myself lucky as the new manager to have such a great group of people to work with and to lead. If it weren't for that one person that dislikes me things at work would be completely perfect!

There's always that one isn't there? That one that distrusts every human being on the face of the planet. That one that will read something negative into your facial expression, rather than assume that you just had an itch run across your brow and scrunched your forehead tightly before rubbing your index finger over your skin. That one that spews venom throughout the genuine and good-natured group of people that you're already proud of even though you just met them. That one that attempts to take you down before you've even risen up to the exciting challenge so recently bestowed upon you. And unfortunately as I enter the building 'that one' is standing at the front of the store with her hands on her hips as she scowls at me for simply walking through the front door.

I smile as if nothing is wrong and greet her with a pleasant 'good-morning.' She squints her eyes and holds her wide mouth in a clamp-like grip, showing no teeth whatsoever as she struggles to respond with a 'good-morning'. She's enraged that I'm even present. She's enraged that the person that used to manage this store has moved on and she gets to meet yet again another store manager. Another store manager that she doesn't know and doesn't trust. She's worried about who I am and what I'm going to do. And the funny thing is that I'm actually the least of her concerns. I'm actually one of those managers that is truly nice! I'm one of those managers that's actually approachable and genuine. And I'm one of those managers that has integrity. If she just relaxes for even a minute she will clearly see that she has nothing to worry about. But that's not the type of person she is. She's more comfortable spewing her venom and flickering her skinny sharp tongue at me as I pass her in my travels to the office. She's coiled into a tight ball of serpentine flesh and she wants nothing more than to strike out at me and plunge her fangs through the flesh on the back of my neck.

"How are you doing this morning?" I'm smiling.

"Fine."

"I'll be right out and we'll hold a quick morning meeting for the team." I'm still smiling.

She says nothing.

Part of me wants to tell her to loosen up and quit with the lousy attitude because if I continue to see examples of her negativity and feel that she's impacting the team in such a manner I will initiate performance management on her ass and work her right the hell out of the building and back through the very front door that I just opened! But I'll hold off on that and give her a chance to come around first. But she'd better hurry up! I'm nice but only to a certain point!

The service desk associate pages 'store manager call on line one' before I even put down my coat and purse. A phone call this early in the morning cannot be good news.

"Hello." I'm sounding like I'm smiling but I'm not at all.

"Have you seen your service result?" It's the boss. He

sounds like he's not smiling.

"Not yet. Why?" I can tell it's bad.

"You have some work to do my dear." I'm his dear? Is this how he talks to the men that are store managers? I can feel the blood in my neck start to boil.

"What was it? Tell me."

"You're the lowest in the district."

"Great." Not great. My boiling blood immediately turns to ice. Ice cold blood is pulsating through my veins on a collision course with my pounding heart.

"What's going on?" He's angry.

"I'm not sure." What the hell does he expect me to say to that question? I'm still new in this store. And I'm at the front of the store kissing ass and babies every single day. And I'm talking with literally hundreds of customers and they love us. I can't see how it is possible in the slightest that the results are poor with our service surveys. This makes no sense whatsoever!

"Well you better figure it out!" Now he's yelling at me.

"I will."

And with that he slams the telephone down. I have tears welling up in my eyes and I'm crossing that bridge from a wooded rural town of uncertainty, over blackened waters, and into a deep thick forest full of doom and destruction! And there are snakes, serpents and reptiles lurking underneath the bridge as I tip-toe across it. They are flickering their tongues and reaching up towards my feet from underneath the rickety wooden bridge with sharp claws and gnashing teeth. They're trying to take me down. They're trying to grab ahold of my ankles so they can whip my body off the bridge, over the rails, and onto the sharp and jagged boulders that line the edge of the swirling blackened waters. They're going to feast upon my dead and lifeless body immediately after my head slams into the rocks. And even if I manage to somehow survive the crossing of the bridge, the fierceness of what lies within the dark forest will surely mean the end of life as I know it! I haven't even finished relocating and I'm already in danger of being fired. I sold my house, am moving my family to a strange and foreign land, and my income is going to be ripped away from me! What have I done??? I'm failing. I'm falling over the edge of the bridge, I'm dying across the jagged edge of the giant boulders and I'm failing my entire family. The room is spinning around me now as I fumble through my desk for a head-piece, radio, my keys, and a daily line-up sheet.

"Let's have a quick team meeting at the front of the store please." I can hear my own voice quivering. I immediately clear my throat and hope that nobody noticed. I need to pull it together. I need to engage this team. The entire team. I need them to understand the importance of what we do and why we do it. I need them to want to do it. I need them to sympathize with our situation and realize that they deserve better results. And I need them to respect me as their leader as I explain all of this to them. But they don't know me yet. They don't trust me still. How in the hell am I supposed to fix this? I need to turn this around.

The entire crowd of ten associates has gathered in a semi-circle at the front of the building. I'm smiling as I welcome them to the day before us. And before I even start speaking to the results of the customer service survey, I invite them to play a game with me.

"Let's start our day off with a game! Who wants to play a game?"

The crowd shifts from being a circle of trepidation to a laughing group of curious onlookers. They're smiling and they're beginning to bounce around. They're loosening up and they're wondering what we're going to be doing. They want to play.

"I'm going to tell you three things about myself. Two of them are true and one of them is not. You have to figure out which is what and the winner gets a prize! And I call this game 'Who's The Manager?' Do you want to play?"

They're all laughing now. The entire crowd is smiling and they are laughing. They are clapping and they are whispering amongst themselves as I begin to tell them the three things about myself that they will need to decipher. And as I talk I'm looking at their bright shiny faces and I'm studying their expressions as I glance from one face to the next around the circle of associates. And then I get to her. I get to that one associate that's still coiled into a tight ball of serpentine flesh as she flickers her skinny tongue in my direction. She's not smiling. She's not laughing. She's standing stiff as a board as she continues to squint her eyes and tighten her mouth. She's growing angrier as the seconds tick by. She wants nothing to do with this game and she wants nothing to do with any efforts whatsoever, on my part, to engage this lovely group of people.

"I love chocolate ice cream." Heads are nodding as I speak. She's just staring.

"I played basketball in High School." They're smiling. Her mouth is tightening still.

"I have a cadaver bone in my body." Now they're laughing out loud. She smirks and shrugs as if to say 'it figures that you're as monstrous as Frankenstein himself!'

As the game continued I found myself calming down. I felt the tears beginning to dry up and I felt that with consistency and persistence I would win the crowd over. They would come to know me as a manager they can rely on, follow and trust. They would begin to do the right thing with and for our customers even if I'm not standing there watching them. They would begin to engage to the tasks at hand and thrive on positive results that they impact for the better of the entire store as well as the customer. They would begin to see me as their leader. Except for her. She's still standing there glaring with her flickering tongue while she spits venom in my direction.

After the game I continued to speak with the team about our results and what we need to do to improve. I watched their expressions as they nodded and listened. They were listening. They were anxious to improve. I felt like I was doing it. I looked around the room and studied each face; one after the other. I could see that they were beginning to become connected. But then I got to her face and she was still just glaring at me. With her tangled dark hair, slit eyes and clamped shut mouth she continued to glare. She was wearing a black blouse, black pants and dark makeup. Everything about her was so dark; except for a tiny piece of something white that was sticking out of her pocket. The tiny piece of something white was a sliver of a visible edge of a small white piece of shiny paper. The kind of paper that receipts are made out of. That tiny little piece of receipt paper was just staring back at me like she was staring back at me with slicing anger. And then it hit me. Why would there be a receipt in her pocket? We weren't even open yet. She hadn't made a purchase. She must have found a receipt on the floor, or in a carriage or somewhere but she had chosen to keep it and slipped it into her pocket for some reason. And the reason should have been as obvious as the horrific results of our customer service score. Every single receipt that we hand to every single customer after every single purchase has a code on it for the customer to enter as they sign onto our website to fill out a survey. And the code is an anonymous code. We, the store associates, have no way of knowing who the customer is when they sign in so they can tell us what they think of us. And the second I noticed the receipt sticking out of her front pants pocket, I immediately darted my eyes straight from the receipt to the deep black pupils in the very core of her irises. And her glare grew even sharper than before as she noticed that I noticed the tiny corner of a bright white receipt peeking from the corner of her pocket. She immediately shoved her hands into both of her front pockets and continued to glare at me. And it hit me. It hit me like a tidal wave of blackened waters surging up and over the edge of the bridge. No wonder the results don't match the efforts I've been making as I continue to kiss ass and shake hands at the front of the store.

Sabotage!

Chapter 10

"Where is this guy's office?"

"Same place as the doctor's office." I'm just staring out the front window of the giant big man car as we drive into Laconia. It's cold out this morning. The off-season rental cottage that we're living in is on a lake. And yesterday morning the water was beginning to thaw. There were dark spots in the center of the lake that suddenly had appeared. And the very edge of the lake was actual water. But when I woke up this morning the entire lake was yet again completely covered with a thick harsh blanket of solid ice. We're moving toward the spring but we're not quite there yet. It's like a heart beating across the thin roll of paper that slides through the electrocardiogram machine. The heart is beating and peaking and dropping in jagged formation. Just when it peaks the ice finally begins to melt, but suddenly the crisp black line that documents the heart's rhythm drops to the very bottom edge of the graph; that's when everything freezes again. That's when the ice returns and overtakes the entire surface of the deep dark lake. And then it changes yet again. Within mere moments the surface of the lake freezes, melts and refreezes over and over again. And the entire community continually slips beneath a huge blanket of the frigid arctic air of a typical New England winter. There is absolutely nothing that any of us can do about it. It will happen over and over again and we are helpless as we jolt and surge with the jagged black ink of the electrocardiogram. And I'm sick of it. And I don't like being cold.

In a few weeks my family and I are going to Puerto Rico! I'll be able to get warm once we get there. And I can't wait! This is my family's third time there. It's an entire family reunion vacation this time though and there are two dozen of us going. We've been planning the trip for two years now. Every two years we have a family reunion vacation. Every two years we travel somewhere together and try to enjoy a week of relaxation and time spent with the extended family. Every two years there's a furious explosion of drama amongst certain family members when we are on vacation. The first ever family reunion was in Virginia. We had rented a cluster of houses on the Chesapeake Bay. The caravan drive all the way from New England to Virginia tested my nerves. Albert's brother led the way and felt he had to pull over at nearly every single rest stop. We would just get things rolling along the highway, just get the kids settled down and he would suddenly be veering down the exit ramp to another rest stop. He needed to go to the bathroom, or get a hamburger, or stretch his legs; one reason after another he would have to stop for another rest. The entire trip took us fifteen hours to get there when it should have only taken eleven. I was ready to commit murder on his ass when we finally pulled into the driveways for the cluster of houses on the Chesapeake Bay.

For the most part it was a great week! We went to Busch Gardens, rode horribly scary roller-coasters, went shopping, went to the beach and found amazing sea glass, and ate a bunch of really delicious food. But when the drama finally hit; the great times and experiences were forever overshadowed by the poor behavior which in retrospect probably isn't poor behavior at all but just typical family bickering. Family bickering that we should probably never give any weight to. Because if you can't misbehave with your family and know that you will always be forgiven and loved unconditionally, then how on earth are you going to release frustrations that build when you find yourself trapped with the extended family for an entire week? It all just needs to be okay. But it wasn't.

One particular sister in-law was and had been enraged with another sister in-law because the second sister in-law hadn't contacted the first when she had found out that the first sister in-law had cancer. Months had gone by, appointments, surgeries, chemotherapy and all the fixings were long since passed with never even a single telephone call. The first sister in-law was never going to get over it and had become somewhat of a bully when she enticed her two daughters to join rebel forces with her and against the second sister in-law. So when the second sister in-law finally asked the first how she was feeling on day three of the family reunion vacation, the room became a boiling pit of inferno's rage and bubbling oil with leaping flames and pitchforks! Thank God I was merely an observer and not a partaker of the effects. It was just another typical family reunion!

"What floor is he on?" Albert and I both scurried from the car through the parking lot and into the warm building as fast as we could.

"Second I think." Without even looking for or asking for directions, I begin to walk up the stairs to the second floor. This facility is so crisp, clean and friendly that I'm not worried at all about finding my way. What's the worst that can happen if I'm wrong and I go to the wrong floor? I need to take another set of stairs?

"Are you sure?"

"No."

"Shouldn't we ask?" Albert's nervous.

"No." I'm not. I open the door which leads to a narrow hall with an opening of offices at the end. There is a waiting room with just a dozen or so orange chairs and paintings of landscapes on the wall. The nurse at the reception desk is pleased to see another patient approaching and greets me with a warm hello and an offer of assistance.

"I'm here to see Dr. Alright." I love the surgeon's name. It makes me feel like it will be just that. I'm still rather perturbed at the idea of even having a 'surgeon' assigned to me. I wonder how much money this office visit will cost me. I'm completely positive that it will be huge given that he is after all a surgeon. I'm sure he charges more than my primary care doctor will for the appointment to take and read the x-ray.

"You can have a seat."

"Okay. Thank you." I smile. How come there's no paperwork? I've never been here. Shouldn't I have to be filling something out? Maybe I don't have to because this is the same medical group and all of the paperwork I filled out for the primary care doctor is quite enough. Maybe they have all of the answers to all of the questions they need? Maybe there's nothing else they need to know? Maybe it's not me that is about to provide any answers; maybe it's going to be the opposite?

Why are there no other people in here? Why aren't all of the chairs full of people that are frustrated beyond reason because they're tired of waiting to see the surgeon? I can hear voices through the walls and through the white door that leads from the waiting room to the hallway full of examination rooms. I know there are other patients in the building. I'll say it again: this medical facility and actually the entire area full of doctors, hospitals, examinations rooms, specialty clinics...they all know how to schedule it right and I just can't believe it! Almost as soon as I sat down, once again, the nurses were right on point and I was called into a small examination room. My God, they are so good at this!

As I pulled myself up and onto the examination table a different nurse from the first one greeted me with pleasantries and took my vital signs. She had bleached blonde hair pulled tightly into a bun and wore a red pair of reading glasses which were teetering on the very tip of her nose. Her eyes were a piercing blue color with eyelashes that were so long, I swear they must be fake. As she continued to chatter about the weather and how she was ready for all of the snow to finally melt away, she opened up my file on the laptop which sat on a swinging arm/table looking thing. Suddenly she became serious as she read whatever information was on the laptop screen and I watched as her expression changed. She stared at the screen on the laptop and then looked at me without speaking, back to the screen, back to me, to the screen and over and over again. She's not talking anymore. She suddenly became quiet and I felt as if I'd walked into a room full of people that immediately stopped talking when they saw me approaching. What is she reading on that screen? What does it say about me? Why is she so quiet all of the sudden? She quickly ended her part of the transaction and exited the room.

"Wonder what that was about?" I'm chuckling as I swing my legs to and fro over the edge of the examination table when suddenly I could feel something inside of me moving. I felt something brewing within my chest. I could feel a tingle of heat beginning to grow and I twisted and turned to see if there was a window that we could open for just a minute.

"It's hot in here."

Albert just stood off to the side leaning against the counter.

"My body is heating up." Suddenly I was becoming a burning pit of molten lava that was erupting from the very depths of my soul. The heat was deep. It was deep and right within the center of my chest. And I knew that was coming. The hair along the underside of the back of my head suddenly felt as if it were sticking to the back of my neck. I could feel tiny little streams of beaded sweat running down the front of my blouse, across the small of my back and down the sides of my rib cage. I was dripping; I was literally dripping with sweat.

"Where the hell is this guy?"

Albert was leaning his head forward and scrunching up his forehead as he looked at me.

The walls of the examination room are covered with posters and pictures of internal organs and artist renditions of the human body. There are cupboards and a sink with a counter that is completely stuffed with jars of wooden sticks, cotton balls and a small tray of shiny examination instruments and things that look like they'd be fun to play with. What the hell are the cotton balls for? I've never seen a doctor or nurse use a cotton ball? When they give you a shot they clean the 'spot' with a packaged alcohol wipe. Then they put a bandage on it. What are the cotton balls for?

"Is there a thermostat in here?" I'm twisting and turning as I pull my hair off the back of my neck. "I should have pulled my hair up." I'm dying! This heat is completely unbearable and I'm going to explode into a thrusting volcanic eruption if the air in this freaking tiny little room doesn't start to move! I can't freaking breathe!

"How are you?" A large man with a goatee swings the door open and reaches out to shake my hand. "I'm Dr. Alright."

Oh thank GOD! The air is moving just a bit from the swinging of the door and it's enough that I caught the very edge of it. I'm fanning myself as he enters and I quickly stop and sit up to full attention.

"Nice to meet you." I'm shaking his hand and I'm trying to read his expression. He's smiling but his eyes look serious. He's making me nervous. I have that feeling again. What the hell is going on in here? Why did they crank the heat up the second I sat on the freaking examination table? What are these people doing to me anyway? I have that feeling that I've been here before but I haven't been here before but I know something is going to happen. What the hell is going on? And how come the doctor isn't hot? He's wearing long sleeves, a tie, and a white medical jacket/coat over all of that. How can he not be melting in all of that clothing? Who the hell are these people anyway?!

"I've looked at your C Scan and there's something there."

Okay, you know what? That's it! Stop right there if you're only going to tell me that there's something there! I already know that there's something there. They told me there was something there when they did the MRI at the Orthopedic Center. They told me there was something there when they took the x-ray. We already know there's something there! You better not just be telling me that once again we have discovered that there's something there! You'd better be getting ready to give me some freaking answers and not just repeating the exact same thing that the other doctors have already told me! You're a freaking surgeon already! You'd better know something! And turn down the freaking heat while you're freaking at it!

"What is it?"

"Let me show you." He immediately pulls the arm/table thing with the laptop and hits an icon on the desktop screen. Suddenly a fuller than life image of my chest is moving, living and breathing across the computer. And as he twists the tiny little knob that sits in the front center of the wireless computer mouse, the image moves. We are traveling through the center of my very core and the image is breathing and moving in dark and white smudges of skin, bone, organs and tissue as we travel. Deeper and deeper we move through my torso and I suddenly feel like I've slipped into a hidden well, that lurked beneath the tall grass and broken branches as I walked along the edge of that little farmhouse I owned years ago in Canterbury, New Hampshire. The house that we used to live in some twenty years ago and the house that I cried about when we left it and moved back to Maine. There was a well that we found one day as we cleaned the perimeter of woods that fenced the huge back yard. An old hand-dug well that hadn't been used since the property farmed cows, chickens and pigs. And innocently as I skipped through the flying fuzz and floating butterflies, I suddenly landed foot first into the deep and dark dirt that sank at least fifty feet below the surface of the earth. And today I've fallen into it. Not just one of my feet has slipped but both of them have fallen through the broken, rotten wooden covering that lays across the opening of the deep, moldy well. And it smells like decay. There is decay all around me. The earth is rotten and it is thick and it is dark. And I'm falling. I'm falling deeper and deeper into the well and I'm screaming for help and I don't even know why!

"Wow." Albert has leaned forward and he is staring in silence at the living and breathing image of my chest.

We're rolling through the image and the edges are moving and twisting and sliding all across the screen. The lights in the room seem to be dimming as we continue to stare at the images of white and black. The air is dank and thick. I feel like I'm spinning as I continue to fall deeper and deeper into the blackness of the hand-dug well along the edge of the Canterbury property. And it's so hot that I can't even breathe. The walls of the well are dripping and I can hear the water as it gathers into a deep pot of boiling, thick liquid full of bacteria and floating dead bodies of tiny rodent like creatures.

"Right there."

He's pointing. Dr. Alright is leaning forward and he's pointing at something that looks like a large bubble of whiteness and thickness on the very edge of the image of my torso. "Do you see this?"

"Yes." Albert speaks first.

"Yes." I repeat what he already said for us both.

"This is the issue." The surgeon turns his head away from the screen and stares into my eyes.

"What is it?" I'm staring. The walls are made of dirt and the ceiling is dripping with a horrific and putrid stench of rot. The slashing heat, which I thought poured through the air conditioning ducts in the examination room is actually rising up from the very bottom of the deep dank well that my body is slipping further into. My blouse is completely sticking to my skin across the small of my back. I lean forward and grab my purse from the chair that sits next to the examination table and start rummaging through it for a hair clip. I have to get my hair off the back of my neck! I can't take the heat anymore!

"Do you see this one too?" He's pointing at the screen as he continues to scroll us through the deepening images of my torso. Another large white cloud that sort of looks like a giant white bubble has formed along the edge of my lung.

I'm slipping. I'm slipping deeper and deeper into the filth and putridness of the dark hand-dug well. I'm trying to grab hold of the sides of the well. There are roots of trees and broken branches and jagged rocks protruding through the walls of the well and my hands keep slapping and grabbing to try and stop myself from sinking deeper and deeper into the darkness and the horrific stench of rotten earth!

"Yes, I see it." I'm rummaging through my purse and I can't see anything. My hands are searching blindly for a large plastic hair clip. But my purse has so much stuff in it! I can't find anything! And the stuff that's in my purse has completely taken over every zippered inside pocket, change purse and makeup pouch. The stuff isn't the stuff that I normally would find inside of my purse and I can't figure out what has happened to the contents that I normally would be searching through right now. My purse is loaded with damp rotten dirt and broken tree roots and chips of bark. My nails are digging through the filth and grime in a desperate search for my hair clip. I need to get my hair off the back of my neck before I vomit all through this freaking examination room. Where the hell is my hair clip! What the hell is happening to me?!

"And then there's another one over here." He's still showing us the findings. He's still scrolling through my torso full of white, black and gray images of flesh, bone and things we can't identify.

I can't breathe. Everything in this room is covered with hot dirt, dripping grime, and the smell of dead decaying rodents. "What is it?" I can't see him. I think my eyes have shut.

"Well, I'm not sure. We need to do a biopsy." Is he even talking to me? He's still staring at the computer screen and scrolling through the images.

"What are we looking for then? Why do we need to do a biopsy?" I can hear the words coming out of my mouth but I sound like I'm a million miles away from what's happening in the small examination room. Dr. Alright turned away from the laptop and now he is just staring at me. I can't even concentrate on the words that are coming out of his mouth. They're echoing through the walls of the dripping, rotten well that I just continue to fall deeper and deeper into. Just say it! Just tell me what you think it is already! You're a surgeon for Christ's sake! You have an opinion don't you? You are looking at the screen and you are pointing at something that is causing enough concern that you want to take a knife and cut into my freaking chest and grab a bunch of cells to shove underneath a microscope don't you? Well...why? What is it??

The heat beneath my feet is burning my soles. I can't see a thing through the darkness and I can feel the sharp broken tree roots along the wall of the well, slash and slice the skin along the very edges of my rib cage as my arms flail wildly above my head. Am I dying? Is this how it all ends? I innocently frolicked along the edge of a property that I loved and for whatever reason failed to see the danger right in front of me. I failed to anticipate what was coming. I failed to follow the correct path. I failed myself. And now I've lost control and I'm just falling.

"With this type of presentation, we are typically looking at mesothelioma."

Everything just stopped.

The air isn't moving.

I'm pretty sure I'm not breathing.

That's the second time somebody used that word.

Albert is just standing there.

I don't know how many minutes passed in silence before I suddenly realized that I was completely and horrifically wedged within the putrid walls of the dank, dark and rotten well. My body has just become completely stuck. One of the jagged edges of the deep hand dug well, has a protrusion of rock, roots and thick dank dirt and my body has become wedged between the protrusion and the other side of the well. The heat is raging beneath my suspended body and I am dripping with the rotten, bacterial infested dew that collects in the pool of blackness at the bottom of the well.

I'm not even sure who spoke first.

I'm not sure what broke the silence that we were all completely immersed within.

I remember dropping my head forward as my lifeless body drooped across the jagged rock protruding through the moldy dirt wall of the deep hand dug well.

I remember crying. And even though I was crying, my tears were indistinguishable from the dripping dew that screeched across my dirt stained cheeks. The entire room was completely silent. The air was so thick that it was impossible to take even a single breath. There was no oxygen. There was no movement in the air whatsoever. It was nothing but complete and utter silence. I remember crying in the silence.

Suddenly Albert was next to me and slowly reached down and lifted my drooping head and laid it gently against his shoulder. And all I could do was cry. I couldn't focus on anything because there was nothing but pure blackness within the deep moldy walls of the hand dug well. I couldn't lift my eyes to see what Albert was doing. I could only feel that he was embracing me. The air was so thick and dank that as much as I struggled I couldn't get a breath. I desperately needed to fill my lungs with cool fresh crisp mountain air. I desperately needed to breathe but I could not. It was as if there were no oxygen whatsoever. And as much as I struggled to take a breath and feel some relief for the horrific pressure across my lungs, I could not force the air to enter my very being and relieve my soul. I heaved and heaved with a horrific guttural sob as my anguish seemed to take over my entire being.

My head slid back down and away from my husband's shoulder and I remember hearing Albert whispering to me with a feeble and quivering voice as he told me that everything was going to be okay.

Chapter 11

Is maxification a word?

I can't help but feel like I have become completely saturated with useless information and zero explanation. And the level of my frustration cannot be described. How is it that I can see three separate doctors, have three separate tests and be left with nothing but 'opinions' up to this point. And it's bothering me that the opinions are all matching for some reason. How can everybody just point to the worst case scenario and actually have the nerve to tell me that they're comfortable saying that I have Mesothelioma when we haven't even had the biopsy yet? How can this be a good process? How does it make sense to connect the fact that 'something's there' to one of the worst forms of rare and somewhat inoperable cancers? Mesothelioma is a death sentence isn't it? I looked it up on-line after the first doctor used that word. And everything I read points to the 'mere six months to live program' which you don't get to decide if you want to be a part of! You just get voted into it! It's like the world decided to hold a secret election. Just prior to the election the world went through an entire list of possibilities and the world nominated a small handful of potential members of the Mesothelioma club. And with no word, question, inquiry, interview or debate you wake up one morning to discover that congratulations are in order! You discover that you are one of the elite few that's been voted into the club!

And at this point I really just need to know what the point is with all of these appointments, conversations and tests if everybody is giving me nothing more than an opinion! I don't need an opinion I need facts! What is the 'something's there' that everybody keeps talking about? What am I paying these experts for? If we saw that there is a 'something's there' when we took the MRI then why did we need an x-ray? If we saw that there is a 'something's there' when we took the x-ray then why did we need the C Scan? If we saw that there is a 'something's there' with the C Scan then why am I hearing again for the third time in a row that the 'something's there' is probably most likely cancerous tumors but it has to actually and specifically be Mesothelioma?? Are we not just repeating the exact same thing through additional testing and opinions over and over again? Am I stuck inside of that movie with Bill Murray?? Every morning I wake up to the same alarm clock song singing through the hotel room, there's a blizzard outside, and Punxsutawney Phil is about to either see his shadow and run or come outside and play.

One of the things I hate most of all is when people come to me with news but they don't know what the news is or what I am supposed to do with the information that they are giving me. So of course when this happens I don't focus on the news at all, I rather decide to instead focus on the incompetence of that individual who doesn't have enough sense to present me with the news AND some answers, details, direction or shred of explanation. And when that individual is a medically trained professional that I am quite literally paying to do a job and tell me what the freak is going on and what the hell am I supposed to do about it, my saturation level of patience reaches its max!

I'm actually quite done. I don't want to hear another word about a single thing from a nurse, doctor, receptionist, or volunteer grandmother at the entrance to the hospital. I want the facts. I need to get my head around what is going on and I need a plan of action. This constant spinning and spewing of identical information and opinions is getting me nowhere other than to the very point I was at when Brad first called. I am quite literally maxxed out!

So at this point the question on my mind: Is maxification really a word? It should be. Because that's the state that I'm in. Is this a stage? Is this the first thing that happens to you when you get horrible medical news and scary words are being tossed throughout the room while you sit on the edge of the examination table and peer down into the horrific dark stench of the Canterbury well? What's the second stage? How many total stages am I going to get to go through and how quickly will I get through them because I am completely sick of the stage that I'm in right now!

Maxification: the complete and utter state of frustration and saturation with the useless and repetitive information coming from medical professionals which you are actually paying to find out and tell you what is wrong with your body, but they can't so they just instead say they are comfortable with the current diagnosis from the first guy at the Orthopedic Center who simply stated: "Something's there."

Chapter 12

It is so quiet in this store. The store that I worked at before 'my store' was so much busier. There was a constant flow of angry looking people and half of them belonged to freaking gangs and the other half pretended and just acted like they wanted to. Many of them yelled at their children that should have been in school but for whatever reason were running around the store as their pissed off mothers shopped for items they 'had to have'. And by the way the children acted, I imagined that they weren't in school because they had been expelled for poor behavior. Behaviors they had most likely learned from the very women that were carting them around the departments while they screamed and swore at them.

What has happened to our society? Where did so much disrespect come from anyway? The way the general public acts is so horrifying and the complete opposite of the way I was raised to act. When I was a little girl and my mother took me shopping I behaved. I grew up learning to "leave things the way you found them" and knowing that if my mother even looked at me cross-eyed, I'd better stop what I was doing immediately! Heaven forbid I heard the comment, "You just wait until your father gets home." Then I was really going to get it! And it was because of these comments and instruction that I always behaved. But this doesn't happen anymore. Somewhere along the way the generations shifted. Probably when mothers had to go to work and could no longer stay home to raise the children properly. Everybody is so busy now. They don't have time to do the good jobs that the mothers of my day did. So they get frustrated. And the more and more frustrated they become, the more they spiral out of control with their own children and their own lives.

"Good morning!" I'm so sweet I'm dripping sugar on the customers that enter 'my store.' My customers seem nice. They smile. Many of them are quite old. Those are the people that I truly want to talk to. Those are the people with the best stories and the best experiences. Those are the ones that remind me of my grandmother.

"How are you?" A little old lady is smiling at me.

"I'm great. How are you doing?"

"I'm cold." She's laughing as she tightens her pink fleece jacket around her neck.

"It is cold out there isn't it?" I'm smiling.

"I have to ask you a question. You're the new store manager aren't you?" Her voice is so sweet and soft sounding.

"Yes. How can I help you?"

"I was in a couple of days ago. When that other manager was working."

"Other manager?"

"You know the one with the black hair?"

"A girl?"

"Yes." She's peering at me through glasses that are so thick they make her eyes look giant.

"Okay." Great. What did that snake do now?

"You know what she told me?" The little old lady's head is quivering. It's bobbing quickly back and forth in tiny little shaking movements. She's so adorable but clearly bothered by something.

"What?"

"She said that you won't let people use coupons here anymore." I think she's going to cry. Clearly she must be on a limited income. Clearly she relies on savings as she shops just like the rest of us.

"She said that? Oh my goodness, no. That's completely untrue. You can use your coupons here anytime." I'm shaking my head as much as the little old lady now. I'm trying to comfort and console her as I explain what a huge misunderstanding we must have.

"She told all of us that. I was here with my daughter and grandchildren. She said that the new store manager told her to stop taking customer coupons."

I wonder if the little old lady could see my blood bubbling through the pulsating veins in the sides of my neck. I wonder if she could tell that as sweet and soft as my voice sounded, beneath is was a furious river of screaming rage. At what depths will the snake sink to? The sabotage is so much deeper than I could have imagined. The snake wants me to be obliterated from the position I have just accepted. She wants me gone. She want me out of here! I think she'd be happy if I just keeled over and freaking died already! In effect what that really means is that she wants nothing more than to just murder me already!

The snake is slithering through the tall grass and hiding as she slinks along her way throughout the deepest corners of the store. She's lurking and she's lashing out. She's plotting her course and she's striking out for my flesh at every opportunity that crosses her path. She wants to poison me with her venom. Venom which will ravage my physical being from the inside to the out. Venom that will cause the rapid decline of my vital organs. Venom that will quite literally burn the skin from around the site of her vicious freaking bite.

Why is she so angry? Why does she want to destroy me? She doesn't even know me. She hasn't even given me a chance and already she's trying to take me down and get me the hell out of this store. And what will she gain by doing that? She's not in line for the position I've been given. She is intelligent enough to know the process within this company. She knows that certain steps are taken before people are given positions and she's taken none of those necessary steps. So even if I were to disappear forever she would not be promoted. Another manager would be coming through the very same doors that my little old lady customer just walked through.

Or maybe she doesn't know the procedures? Maybe she's been lied to? Maybe she's been told that she's getting this store time and time and time again; yet she continues to see complete strangers get promoted while she sits in the wings waiting and waiting and waiting for nothing that ever comes? Maybe it's not that I'm here at all? Maybe it's that the person that used to be here is gone? Maybe that's truly the issue. Maybe the anger that burns within her very core isn't personal at all; how can it be? She doesn't know me.

Yet still the snake remains. It lurks and it lingers in the shadows of the store that I've come to call my own. And she's waiting for that perfect moment. She's building her bed of broken promises to our customers, sabotaged survey results, and traps that she's setting. And she's watching with her slits for eyes, clamped shut mouth and flickering tongue.

"I'll always take your coupons." I'm still smiling at the

elderly customer.

"Oh good!" She's smiling. "I knew you would."

My customers are nice.

The snake should go to work at the store that I used to work at before coming to this one. She'd fit right in there. She's definitely a city snake!

Chapter 13

"Oh crap." That was the text I received from my boss when I texted him and told him that I needed a day off for the biopsy.

"Keep me posted." That was the second text I received.

And I can just imagine what he must be thinking right now. I just got here. He just hired me. And I haven't even begun to get my hands and head around my new role, who the team is, what this community is about, and what kind of new store manager I am truly going to be and now I'm sick…potentially. Potentially I'm the kind of sick that will in all likelihood cause me to need to be out of work for a period of time if not forever. 'Oh crap' is right! He doesn't even know me. And I feel like I've wasted his time. Does 'Oh crap' indicate that he's actually worried about me and my family or does 'Oh crap' mean that he's irritated that the store will potentially be without a manager? If 'Oh crap' means that it's all about me and my potential illness, then perhaps 'Oh crap' would never have existed because he would rather have called me directly instead. And it's probably evil of me to even think that about this man but the fact of the matter is that I don't know him either.

"Where do we go?" Once again Albert and I are driving the giant big man vehicle into the town of Laconia.

"The hospital." I don't want to go. This is stupid. This is another waste of time. I don't care what they are telling me about their opinions. They are wrong! My shoulder was just hurting! That was all this was! Now I get to have a useless procedure and when I even think about it, it is making me sick to my stomach! And when it's over and they tell me that there's nothing wrong I'm going to be mad! When that surgeon comes into the examination room, in a couple of days when we get the results, he's going to say 'I guess that's just the way your body looks. There's nothing there after all! It looked like a tumor but in fact it's not. How about that?' And he will be smiling. And I will stare at him with disdain and complete and utter rage because he is wasting my time and my money! And the procedure will have hurt!

"Where in the hospital?"

"No idea."

"Where should I park?" He's spinning the car through the crazy parking lot. And as much as I should be focusing on the medical procedure I'm about to have instead I decide to take out my rage with the situation on the design of the parking lot. It's an easy target. It's a target I'm familiar with. It already bugs me. "Who the hell designs these freaking things?"

"What?" Albert's just not in touch with my brain right now.

"The parking lot! It's so stupid! There's only one way out and one way in. And if you don't know that and you're trying to maneuver your way around to find a decent parking spot you get sucked all the way into the back of the thing, where the only people that park there are the people that work at the hospital. And when you continue to try and fight your way around the long rows of cars that point one way and then another, eventually you find that you've gone way too deep and now you can't even spin around. You're stuck! You're stuck trying to wiggle back and forth and back and forth until you've managed to turn the HUGE car around, so you can fight to get back out, so you can start all over again and just try to find a freaking parking spot!"

"There's one." Albert's staring at me. "This is close enough to the entrance I guess." I can hear his voice shaking. He's nervous. What the hell is he nervous about? It's not like he has to get a freaking knife shoved into his lung. I'm the only one that has the right to be nervous right now!

"I can't believe this is out-patient. This is going to hurt!" I take a big cleansing breath but it totally does nothing for me.

Albert says nothing. We park and scurry through the cold crisp morning air. It's the kind of cold that actually makes it feel like the tiny hairs in your nostrils freeze with the first inhalation that you take when exiting a warm car or house. I don't like it. And why isn't Albert talking? In fact why did he even come with me? He keeps grunting and groaning like he is physically uncomfortable. And with every little noise that he makes as we walk into the hospital I am growing more and more irritated with him. He acts like he's eighty years old. He acts like he ran a marathon yesterday and his body is sore and trying to desperately recover. Marathon my ass! I'm pretty sure when I got home from work his ass was still sitting on the ugly couch in the off-season rental cottage, in his bathrobe, with the freaking remote in his hand!

"Where do we go?" Albert is spinning around like a toddler that's lost his mother in a busy shopping mall. Now I'm just going to have to completely ignore him. If I don't ignore him I'm going to kill him. I'm going to kill him right here in the front of the lobby, in front of witnesses that don't deserve to be exposed to such a horrific scene of rage and frustration with the fact that the parking lot is completely insane and not only is my husband lost, even though we just walked through the front door but he also can't seem to take one freaking step without grunting, groaning and making an entire series of freakishly weird noises! It's like he has Tourette's Syndrome or something very similar!

"Good morning. I'm here for a biopsy but I'm not sure where I should go." I'm smiling at a nice little old lady that's sitting behind the information desk at the entrance. Albert is still spinning in circles. I should ask the lady if she has any helmets for my disturbed husband who eventually will become dizzy from the spinning and fall to the shiny tiled floor, on which he most assuredly will smack his big head! And immediately all attention will be shifted to him because he will have cracked open his freaking skull unless we get a helmet onto it! Just like when I delivered every single one of our five children! He fainted! He fainted and fell right over and onto the freaking floor. And I'm lying there on the delivery table, surrounded by doctors and nurses when all of the sudden they leave my ass there trying to push out a baby, so they can shove smelling salts underneath Albert's freaking nose because his feeble little ass just fell over and onto the hard tiled floor! He's such a dick-head!

"Go right through that entrance to your left and check in with the desk." She's smiling.

"Thank you." That was easier than I expected. I can hear Albert shuffling and grunting behind me as I march onward and through the doors to the 'unknown but I just know it's going to hurt section' of the hospital. Albert sounds like he can't breathe. And maybe that's the problem. Maybe he just can't breathe. Maybe he's just continued to gain pound after pound since the day we were married and all of the added weight is just pressing up and against the bottom of his rib cage causing his lungs to be unable to fully expand. So now when he even tries to walk behind his wife, through the hallways and corridors of a hospital he is forced to grunt, groan and snort as he struggles to breathe and keep up with her pace! He really needs to just lose some freaking weight already! Or maybe just get off the couch, put down the bag of chips and get a freaking job! That might help with the weight!

The waiting room is completely empty. There's literally hundreds of magazines on multiple tables and in multiple magazine holders but they are perfectly neat. They look as if nobody has touched them, like ever. Like this is the grand opening of the waiting room and not a single person has sat in a chair, picked up a magazine and looked at the beauty ads while flipping pages over and over and over while waiting to be called in for a medical procedure that's going to hurt.

I immediately choose a seat next to one of the small tables with neat magazines. Albert seemed to fall into his chair next to mine and right away begins to rub his knees. How is it that a few months ago he had one knee swell up (which oh by the way he would have ignored if it weren't for me TELLING him to go to the doctor) and now all of the sudden the story he's begun to tell is that he needs a double knee replacement? This is what he's graduated to within his mind. This is totally the story that he tells people now! Complete strangers as well as his own family members. I hear him say things like 'both my knees are shot.' What the hell is he talking about? And if they are hurting him so bad that he has to suddenly shuffle along, fall into his chair and immediately rub them while he groans out loud, then get your ass to a freaking doctor already! And oh by the way, 'your knee was just fine yesterday!' Who's the show for right now anyway? There's nobody in this waiting room except for me! And if he freaking thinks that he's getting sympathy from me right now as I try to mentally prepare myself for the procedure that's about to happen to my own freaking self, he's completely crazy and better get his ass back to the lady at the information desk and beg her for that helmet that we should have asked for! Because he no longer needs to worry about slipping and falling from dizziness and cracking his skull; he needs to be worrying that I'm going to freaking crush it!

"You can come in now." A pretty nurse is standing in the doorway, waving at me.

"Okay." I immediately and very quickly stand up and walk away from Albert without even acknowledging the fact that he's still groaning and rubbing his knees.

"Do I stay here?" Albert's stopped groaning and rubbing for a mere moment as he asks the question.

"Yeah. You stay here." I'm angry. I'm marching. I'm not looking back at him. I never even turn to the nurse to ask if my husband can in fact come with me because I feel that the answer would most assuredly be no; plus I'm so completely aggravated with my situation that I just cannot be around anybody right now. I need to get through this but I don't want to. I don't know what to expect. I don't know what I'm supposed to do. I don't know why this is happening to me. I look into the eyes of the pretty nurse who obviously recognizes my confused expression. She's met me before. I was the other patient that she had on a different day, at a different time, for a different procedure but I was exactly the same person as me.

"We're going right down the hallway to your right." She's walking so softly I think she's floating across the surface of the shiny tiled hallway. I don't even think she has any feet. There's a long flowing dress that wisps around in all different directions where there should be a pair of ankles attached to where there should be two feet in high heeled shoes or clogs that clomp and clomp throughout the halls as she guides the many patients that walk through the door. Where are her feet? And what is up with the very bottom edge of the dress that is forever spinning in circles around her invisible ankles like a cat that wants attention from the owner that's just come through the front door of a tiny little house at the end of Mulberry Drive?

There's music playing. I can hear soft melodies chanting behind the door at the end of the short hallway that the nurse is guiding me through. The music sounds like a ballet or some sort of play or something. It's not music that I hear on the radio. It's more like a classical sort of music. And it's calming. But I'm not calm.

"Come right into this changing room. Take everything off and put on a Johnny. Place your clothes in the locker, take the key with you and come back out." She's still smiling as she holds the door to a tiny changing room open for me.

Without a comment I smile at her and follow the complete instruction. My mind feels like mush and I have shifted gears. I am no longer focusing on rage toward my poor husband who's probably sitting in the waiting room more confused than I am. He gets no direction or answers; he just gets to wait. My mind has suddenly shifted to a complete and utter loss for any explanation so I'd better just stare straight ahead and do what 'they' tell me to do. I don't know what is happening and I can't seem to comment on anything. I'm just obliging every command that I receive. I'm following the directions. I'm focusing on my breathing which seems to have become extremely deep and shallow. My entire world has become the sound of deep raspy breaths that are underneath the crushing weight of an entire ocean. I'm staring straight ahead without a single drop of an emotion. I'm staring and I'm breathing and that's completely it. I think I just became a freaking zombie or something.

As the nurse continues to float and smile, I just trudge and stare and breathe. I'm an empty shell that breathes and trudges after her. I must have split personalities and the one that I've known for my entire life has just been taken over by this strange and completely lost personality that is truly nothing more than a total and complete zombie. I have just crossed over a bridge from one stage of survival mode, into another stage which will help me to cope with the tragedy so recently bestowed upon me. I have no understanding of what is going on around me. First it was Maxification and now I'm barreling through stage two: Zombification! I'm merely existing as I continue to trudge from the tiny changing room, back into the hall, across the way just a few more steps and into a large room with a team of waiting experts standing around a huge machine.

For some reason I feel like the team of experts is excited to see me. They're all smiling and they are bouncing up and down. It's like I'm a zombie rock-star! It must be somewhat rare that the team of experts in this particular hospital gets to perform this type of procedure. It's not like we're at one of the really big hospitals in Boston, Massachusetts. It's not like this is what they do every single day. So when I aimlessly trudge my way through the doors, with my head lopping off to the side, drool dripping down my chin, skin that's turning a pale-gray-green color, and absolutely no noise whatsoever except for my rasping deep shallow breaths, they are undoubtedly excited to see me. They would have paid money for the tickets to this show and they all have a role to play as they situate my body on a large cold table that will slide into the giant machine, with a guided missile of a needle and long skinny stick with a sharp moving beak on the end.

"Come right over here and lay on your belly." A handsome young man is stretching out his arm and showing me the way.

Do zombies have bellies? Shouldn't he have said 'come smash your face into this pillow, crush your breasts onto this cold metal surface and try not to drool all over the place'?

Under normal conditions if a nice handsome young man asked me to come lay down, I'd at least giggle as my mind fantasized about a HOST of situations that I could attach to that one request! But none of that happens. My zombie being just stares straight ahead as my zombie body plops forward without even a smile and hoists my lifeless limbs and torso onto the cold metal bed that slides into the giant machine.

"Do you want a blanket?" A young girl is smiling as she tries to help me get comfortable.

"Let's get her a blanket." Another voice answers for me.

"First we're going to give you a local anesthetic."

"Here's a blanket."

"That should warm you up." Somebody giggled.

"Does anybody have a pen?"

"Mark the area."

I can feel fingers running over my back. They're feeling for the bones beneath my skin. Underneath my shoulder blade they are pressing in and trying to find a certain path. They are going to need to go deep. The needle will somehow have to maneuver beneath my shoulder blade and in between ribs before plunging into the tumors as they rest against my right lung.

"Mark it there."

"You're going to feel some pressure."

Holy shit, are they doing it right now? Just like that they're going to stab me with those long sharp things? I can't feel a thing. I feel like they're pressing something into my skin but there's no pain.

"We're going to slide you into the machine now."

Is there something sticking out of my back? Are they leaving me lying across this cold metal table, with zombie drool running across the pillow case, and a large sharp stick of some sort sticking up in the air and out of my back?

Lots of footsteps are running to the other side of the room. The team of zombie-rock star fans has just run into the tiny glass protected closet that sits in the corner of the room of the giant big machine that my body is now sliding forward and into.

Lots of footsteps are approaching me again.

"Okay. We're going to insert the tube now."

That wasn't a tube before? What was the first thing they inserted? I felt something but I can't see it. I don't know what they're doing! And for some reason I have no freaking voice! I have nothing but zombie drool and raspy breathing!

"Try not to move."

Are they kidding? I can't move! I'm too terrified! I'm frozen! I'm a frozen zombie rock star! I can hear them breathing. They are all close to me and they are breathing literally across my back. They are all hyperventilating. They are way too excited about this! My eyes are completely open but I can't see a thing and I can't stop drooling across the pillow that I've buried my face into. Is this what people go through when they've been abducted by aliens? Is this how they feel as they lie on a cold metal table with a thin blanket that's just popped out of a microwave oven and is covering just half of their body? And a team of people, things or aliens are running their fingers over their skin and they're discussing how deep to send the probe into the zombie body?

"Here we go."

SHIT! Now I can feel something! I'm feeling immense pressure! I feel like they're shoving a long thin sharp knife deep into my back. Are they stabbing me?! What the hell are they doing? I thought they were giving me a local? Didn't somebody say something about a local shot of anesthesia? Where did that go? And what the hell was it supposed to do? How come I can feel this? What the hell was the local for? That shit ain't working at all!

All of the zombie-rock star fans are running back to the little room again. They're watching the screen to see how close the long thin metal probes have gotten to the 'something's there' tumor thing that's lurking within my ribcage. Why do they all keep running into that closet? What the hell are they doing? Are they inserting the long sharp stick things into my body an inch at a time and then they all run back to the closet to watch on an x-ray television screen and see if they are following the right path? Shouldn't somebody be the driver? Shouldn't there be like one person that is constantly moving and guiding the long sharp stick things while the rest of them observe? Are they doing that? There must be at least one person sitting next to me as I continue to slide into and out of the machine with the metal rods, and needles sticking out of my back. There must be somebody that is near to me in case I need immediate help. Right?

"Okay. You're going to feel some pinching."

Thank God! There's a voice next to me. It must be the driver. The driver who is actually the maneuverer.

"Ready?"

Is he talking to me or the zombie rock star fans? What am I supposed to be ready for? What does ready mean? Am I supposed to be doing something special now? Or am I supposed to be 'readying' myself for some sort of horrific pain??

Suddenly there was a sound from within my body which sounded like it was metallic snapping of some sort. But I don't think anybody else could hear it. I think it was completely internal. Like when you suddenly can hear your heart beating throughout your entire brain for some reason. Or when you've been swimming under water for too long, you're heading toward the surface and you can hear nothing except for your own gulping of the air that's already lodged within your lungs. Nobody else can hear the noises in your body except you. And that's what I'm hearing right now. And with every single snapping metallic noise within my body, I feel it. I feel the feeling that a piece of my body is being sliced away. A tiny piece of my body is being cut with every loud metallic snap. And even though the pieces of my body that are being cut and taken away, perhaps sucked away within the tiny long sharp tube with a beak on the end, are small; the pain is not. The pain is surprisingly very large. And it's sharp. Sharp like the beak on the end of the long sharp stick thing that is still protruding out of my back as it continues to be driven into the 'something's there' by the maneuverer.

"Oh God." I closed my eyes. Its pitch black in here.

"Breathe."

I can't breathe. Who's he talking to. Zombies don't have to really breathe anyway do we? Aren't we already dead!?

"Breathe."

Chapter 14

"How'd it go?"

"Horrible."

"Are you okay? What happened?"

"Can we just leave and I'll tell you about it in the car?" Just shut up Albert. Don't talk to me. Just shuffle after me as I march through the cold shiny tiled hallways, back toward the entrance which is now an exit from the beautiful hospital with lots of glass windows.

I can hear his groaning and grunting as he once again attempts to be at the center of everybody's universe. He's hoping for some sort of 'are you okay?' from a complete stranger. Then in his mind he can feel as if he's the one that's suffering so his wife doesn't have to. In some way it will make him feel like the one that is taking the brunt of the suffering for the family. He will feel like a protector in some way if he is the one that is in the most pain and refuses to do anything about it so all of the family's focus can be on his poor wife and her medical issues. It's like he's attempting to be a martyr of some sort. What he seems to have forgotten, or perhaps never knew, is that most martyr's end up being persecuted or publically murdered. They are tortured because they refuse to denounce. What the hell is Albert refusing to denounce? And how long is he going to continue with his 'poor me' exaggerations before I ultimately decide that I should be the one to end his misery once and for all? My God, he must have driven his poor mother crazy as a child!

And maybe his knee or knees really do hurt. Maybe he is truly suffering. Maybe the pain just suddenly became excruciating the moment his wife had a surprise and scary medical 'issue' show up. And maybe the fact that I have never seen him acting like he's in so much pain from freaking shifting his body, walking, sitting, standing, breathing, before today is just a weird coincidence. Whatever the case…I DON'T CARE!

"So what happened?"

I slowly turn my head and glared at my husband as we both settled into the front seats of the giant big man vehicle. His eyes are wide and his mouth is hanging open. His hands are resting across the top of the steering wheel and the motor is softly humming in the background. And I thought about whether or not I wanted to try and describe the entire procedure in detail so he perhaps would be able to grasp for just a mere moment what I am truly going through. It's not just about the medical stuff. It's about the fear that accompanies it. It's about the horrific stage of 'zombification' that I have fallen into. It's about the fact that I know nothing about what is going on, can't seem to get any answers about what exactly I have and what I need to do about it, so I can just get through whatever it is that is happening to me. And the whole time I am struggling to gain some sort of understanding for something that just honestly has no logical explanation whatsoever, I am blindly following instruction from people that I've never even met before. People that are excited to see me because of the rarity of the procedures not because they are invested in me as a person. And apparently I'm supposed to trust all of these people with my well-being, even though they are complete strangers to me. I don't even know their names and I have to trust them to take care of me. Because what choice do I have otherwise?

I don't know what to do. My head is hanging sideways, my eyes are staring straight ahead and the only words I seem to have are the ones raging through my mind. The ones that are repeating themselves over and over in my head as a pulsation of pain continues to beat in the center of the right hand side of my back!

"Well?" Albert's still innocently staring at me. He has no idea what I've just come through and he has no idea that for the entire morning I've been secretly screaming at him within the fragile walls of my brain.

I'm struggling. I'm struggling to form the only explanation I can present to my poor innocent husband who really wants nothing more but to know that I'm going to be okay. He wants to know the answers as much, if not more, than I do and he wants to know what just happened to me as he sat in the waiting room grunting and rubbing his freaking knees. Slowly I opened my mouth and tried to speak. I tried to tell him what happened just now. I tried to tell him of the terror within my being and that I was stuck in some sort of parallel world and had morphed into a complete full blown freaking zombie and I didn't know how to find my way back to the world that I thought I lived in just a few short weeks ago!!! I could hear the deep rasping of my breath and I could feel a tiny river of cold drool running down my chin as the words finally came.

"It hurt!"

Chapter 15

Two more days and I get the news about the 'something's there'. Two more days and Albert and I will travel back over to the surgeon's office in the giant big man vehicle and maneuver through the crazy parking lot before running through the cold crisp air and into the medical building.

But today is all about our home! Today is the day that we sign on the dotted line and are handed keys to our new home!

"I can't believe how quickly we're closing on this one!" I'm practically bouncing in my seat as Albert drives the giant big man vehicle into the quaint little town that in an hour or so will be our new home. It will be the place we say we're from, live, and hopefully love! But even though we are closing today, we won't be moving into our new home for another week or so. We need to clean, paint, and install some quick flooring before that big day is finally here. It's easy for me to call it 'quick flooring' because I'm not the one that will be installing it; Albert is. He's a general contractor. He's a mechanic. He's a real estate broker. He pretty much does everything. And for him to install new carpeting in all of the bedrooms and hardwood floors in the hallways, is just like another day at the office (store) for me. And AFTER all of the stuff gets done to our new home then Albert also gets to be the one that drives back to Massachusetts to unload our belongings into a moving truck, drive it up here, unload the truck and turn around and do it all over again. It will take two or three trips to get all of our stuff into our new home.

"We need to go to the bank." Albert is focused on today.

"Where is the bank?"

"Guilford."

I'm not as certain as Albert is about the location of the bank but accept that he knows what he's talking about. While I'm at work he's had more time to drive around, explore and get a good sense of direction.

Within mere minutes we have arrived at the bank, gotten our bank check, and are pulling into the parking lot at the real estate office located right in the center of Laconia.

"So far so good!" I'm literally skipping my way into the office. I'm ready for this. I'm so tired of living out of a suitcase and I need some GOOD news in my life right now! I just want the key. I want to get the key, drive across town, walk through my new house that's completely empty, dusty and dirty, and scream at the top of my lungs that I have a home again!

Quickly we walk into the receptionist area of the office and are greeted by the 'office person'. I still don't know what to call her and I smile politely as I say hello. "Good morning." I barely get the words out of my mouth and the listing broker is suddenly right behind Albert and me.

"Hey! How you guys doing?" And there he is. A large burley man with a New Jersey accent holds out his hand and grins from ear to ear.

"Hello." Albert shakes his hand.

"Come on in and let's do this!" He's happy to be rid of this property. He's happy that he can finally collect on a bank foreclosure that he undoubtedly fought and fought for reduction after reduction on. He wants to get paid.

And I'm shocked that nobody else snapped this property up! And as soon as we signed the papers, I asked the broker why he thought nobody had fought to get this house before us.

"They all needed financing and when you are financed the banks require you to hold flood insurance on waterfront properties. Even though the waterway in front of your house is controlled by the city dam and ain't ever going to flood, the banks expect people to pay eight thousand dollars a year for flood insurance. I had the house under contract a dozen times and each time the deal fell apart because of flood insurance." He's smiling as he shakes his head and waves his arms in the air.

"Seems ridiculous to expect people to purchase something they don't even need!" I laugh out loud.

"Tell me about it!" He snorts when he laughs, which makes all three of us laugh even more.

And just like that we were home owners again! The entire transaction took no more than five minutes, three signatures and the passing over of a large check for two shiny golden keys.

"Let's celebrate!" I'm bouncing in my seat again, as the

giant big man vehicle pulls out of the parking lot.

"We will! As soon as we go check it out!" Albert is more excited than me as we shoot across town to run through our new empty, dirty, dusty home and scream.

I can't help but question why this purchase has been so easy. Why are we here? Why did this house just fall right into our laps? We are supposed to be here. This is exactly how things are supposed to be happening to me and my family right now. I don't know what the outcome is going to be and I don't know how long it will take to figure it out but for some reason I know there's something that is coming and the stage is being set.

As we pull the giant big man vehicle into the driveway of our new home I can feel the hairs on the back of my neck standing up.

Chapter 16

"Can I talk with you?" One of my department managers is standing in the doorway to my office and raps on the side of the open door as her voice trembles. Why is she nervous?

"Sure you can talk to me. What's up?" I'm smiling as I stop typing on the computer.

Immediately she enters my office, kicks the kick-stand at the bottom of the door and closes it, and sits down in one of the three chairs across the front side of my desk.

"I need to tell you about something that's being said about you in the store."

"Okay." I'm crossing my brow now but oddly still smiling. I feel myself cocking my head to the side and for a second I worry that I might be resembling my Yorki-Poo puppy.

"People are talking about that they've heard that you are planning to fire five or six people, you won't let customer's use their coupons, and you actually have a list. Sort of like a hit list of people that you don't like." She's actually got tears in her eyes.

Unfortunately, but maybe not, my reaction is to burst out laughing. I literally fell back in my chair, tossed my head back and busted a gut laughing out loud! Now I was the one with tears in my eyes. "You must be joking right?" This CANNOT be a serious conversation. The girl sitting in my office is sort of a jokester and must be breaking the ice of our conversation by telling a whopper. I'm the nice manager. I'm the manager that store associates cry about when they hear I'm moving on and away from the world we've shared for just a short period of time. I'm the one that buffers and protects the team from the evil lurking snakes and horrific managers that I've worked for in the past. This MUST be a ridiculous prank and she thought if she threw in the most recent rumor that the snake had spread, about me not taking customer coupons, that it would give validity to the joke. She is so clever!

"I'm not joking." She's still got tears in her eyes and she's wiping them away as she chuckles and stutters through the embarrassment she must be feeling as she shares this news with me.

"Seriously?" Still waiting for her to break into a fit of laughter.

"Seriously." She's shifting in her seat.

"What did you say again? I need to hear this one again. I must have heard you wrong. I've already heard the ridiculous rumor that our CUSTOMERS also heard...that I won't accept coupons anymore; which would actually probably get me fired if I ever were to do something as ridiculous as that. Corporate decides what we do and don't do for our customers; not me. But what were those other two things you just said?" I'm leaning forward in my chair and have perched my chin across the top of my folded hands. This should be good. And my biggest challenge right now will be to not interrupt the story with any explosions of anger. And when I say the word explosion, it's not really like an explosion. It's more like the 'Mommy Voice' comes out. The voice that told all of my children over the years that they were in trouble. The voice that told them if they didn't stop what they were doing, start doing something, or asked them for some sort of logical explanation or else they would be in super big trouble. The voice that told them they didn't have to worry about their father, because he would only be angry with them. The voice that told them that Mommy was MAD! The girl sitting in my office is the messenger. She's the one that's trying to help. I need to stay calm even though I can feel my blood beginning to boil.

"Somebody started a rumor and has told every single person in the store that you intend to clean house. She's told them that you are firing a number of the department leads and she said that you actually have a ... she called it a hit list." She's so serious. She's repeating the facts. And she's repeating the facts to me privately and in my office because she knows. She knows that it's a lie. She knows that I'm not that type of person. And she wants to believe what she knows. She wants to believe what she knows because she also must have suffered from a venomous snake attack. She must have been innocently walking through the back of the Home Department in the store when suddenly the lights went down. It must have been after the store had closed. All of the customers were gone and most of the associates had already left the building. And she suddenly must have worried that she needed to hurry to the lounge and retrieve her personal belongings and get out of the building before it was locked. And she quickly began to scurry across the long back wall of the store. And as she scurried she must have started to hyperventilate as her fears grew and grew that she would surely find herself stuck in the building for the night. And suddenly, out of nowhere, the heavy coiling body of the vicious serpent swung from the rafters and struck. It swung and it reeled back its wide open mouth before plunging forward and striking out at her innocence. In doing so it drove its filthy dagger fangs deeply into the vein on the side of her neck and it filled her innocent being with poison. And she's still recovering. She's spent weeks, months and maybe years hiding from the snake as it continues to lurk in the shadows. Waiting and watching for yet again another opportunity to strike out against its innocent victim. And now she sees a chance. A chance that the new manager will not allow the snake to prey on the weak. A chance that the new manager will destroy the evil in the building and no longer stand by and watch as the frightened associates hide and occasionally writhe in pain from yet again another horrific attack.

"How do you know this all to be true?" I'm so calm.

"She told me herself."

"And there are others that have also been told these lies?"

"Yes."

I take a moment and I pause. I'm smiling with my mouth shut and I'm nodding my head as I look at the now calm associate who is immediately relieved at my reaction. As I look at her and think, I am developing my plan. I've done this before. In my many years of store management I've actually seen and done it all. Anything from opening a brand new store, to closing a bad one. At one point in my career I was the manager that was sent to help fix situations with store teams at different locations. On one particular occasion I moved into a hotel and lived down the road from the problem store for an entire month. My job was to figure out what the problems were with the unengaged team, develop a solution, get the ball rolling with the solution, and maintain every single employee in the process. I'm very good at fixing things. I'm very good at building teams. This is why the particular employee sitting in front of me has come to me. It's obvious.

With all of the goodness and reparations for a team, there are some things that I will absolutely not tolerate, however. There are certain things that people do that I will quite simply not allow. Some of these things are the obvious things, such as stealing, never showing up for their shifts, or threatening a customer or fellow associate. Those types of situations really require no thought whatsoever. Those types of situations really amount to nothing more than a termination. But the situation that the employee sitting in my office has brought me is a bit more involved. This type of situation requires a little bit of homework and gathering, if you will, of certain details of the alleged actions. This type of situation needs a plan. A well thought out, all of the T's crossed and I's dotted, plan. Because the ultimate result of this plan will mean that she will be obliterated! Removed! Fired! Gone! The snake will never be allowed to slither through the back recesses of the shadows in the back of the store. She will be forced from the building, across the parking lot, through the field and back into the dark and dangerous woods that she came from. She can return to live with the other dangerous creatures in the woods where she will no longer be just the predator. Once back in the woods she will also become the prey! She will become the prey and she will have to experience the very terror that she herself has bestowed upon the innocent associates. She will learn what it is like to be tortured because she herself will be hiding from the vicious unforeseen attacks by the 'larger than her beasts' that live within the dark and dangerous woods.

"I'm going to need you to send me an email. This email will need to include everything you just told me. This email needs to contain quotes of what she's said to you. Dates and times of when she said these things will need to be included. Do you understand?" I'm nodding my head as I look at my employee.

"Yes."

"I need you to do this right now. You can use my computer. I'll close the door so you won't be disturbed. Okay?"

"Okay."

Quietly I stand up and motion for the girl to sit at my desk. I open up the email program and tell her to call me if she needs anything, as I'll be right outside the door.

"Oh. And I'll also need the names of the other people that she's spoken to." I'm smiling as I look back at her.

"Okay." She's happy now. She's smiling with her eyes.

She knows I will protect her. She knows the snake's days are numbered.

And as I close the door I couldn't help but smile myself. I'm smiling because I'm beginning to build a cohesive team. A team that only wants what is right. They want what is right for themselves and what is ultimately right for the success of the entire team and the store itself. And the funny thing is that the rumor from the snake included that the new manager had a plan for getting rid of people. What started out as a complete and utter lie has suddenly become the absolute truth but that truth will only be delivered unto the vicious tongue flickering snake. The snake has ultimately done the damage to herself.

Chapter 17

I am so nervous! I'm sitting in the front seat of the giant big man car as Albert drives us across town to the surgeon's office to get the results of the freaking biopsy that freaking hurt like shit! In fact it still hurts! Why does it still hurt? When we got home that day and I pulled up my shirt and asked Albert to check and see how the wound looked, he responded with, 'that's it?' And he responded with 'that's it?' because the wound was literally nothing more than what looked like an injection site! An injection site! How can something that small cause so much freaking pain??!! And if the site is so small then it stands to reason that the sharp biting beak on the end of the tube/stick thing was equally as small if not even smaller. How can it still hurt? Are our bodies designed that the deeper we probe the more intense the pain can get? Are the nerves on the inside of our bodies like super bionic nerves when compared to the nerves on the surface of our skin? Are bodies designed that way on purpose so we won't probe, stab, or cut too deeply because we can't tolerate the pain? I'll bet that's it.

"I can't wait to just get this over with." I'm repeatedly breathing deeply and sighing with a long outward breath. I must appear to be readying myself for a big race, as I'm hopping up and down at the starting blocks.

"It'll be fine. There's nothing wrong with you." As Albert talks he smirks his lips which actually annoys me somewhat. I know he's just nervous and the way he deals with being nervous is to excuse the fears. It's somehow easier for him to deal with potential impending doom if he keeps telling himself that there's nothing wrong. And the hysterical part is that if it were him the tides would change. If it were him he would have already called the planet to inform them of his funeral arrangements. But I accept that he processes differently and try to calm my anger over his smirk that seems to just keep saying, 'oh please…stop wasting my time with this.'

"I know. I still think the whole thing is just so freaking stupid. I just want to hear them say it!"

Finally we pull the giant big man car into the crazy parking lot and I swear the drive over this morning must have taken an extra twenty minutes for some reason. And even though we're still early I rush up the stairs, down the hall and into the surgeon's office. I'm always early. Albert is not. But he's pretty good about keeping up with my demands when we are going someplace together. I'm not comfortable if I'm not early. He's not comfortable if I'm not comfortable. It works.

"I have an appointment with Dr. Alright." I still love his name. The girl at the desk is just as pleasant as she was the first time I saw her. She types and types as she stares at the computer screen and she smiles the whole time she is doing it.

"Is it still cold out there?"

"Wicked cold; I think it was ten degrees out when we got up this morning." I'm still shivering even though it's got to be seventy-five degrees in the medical building.

And then it happened. I stood there waiting for a response and she said nothing. I expected her to say something like, 'where do you live?' or 'wow…it was twelve degrees at my house'…or something like that. But she said nothing. She said nothing as she stopped typing and just stared at the computer screen. And suddenly her smile was gone. She looked scared and nervous for some reason. It was like she had frozen solid because we were talking about how cold it was. For a moment I actually wondered if she had slipped into a catatonic sort of state of mind. Does she do this often?

"You can have a seat."

"Thank you." I looked at Albert who stood quietly next to me and he simply said 'what?' He didn't see it.

"Nothing."

I swear thirty seconds later we were beckoned by a little old lady nurse to come with her through the door and into the hallway of examination rooms. I didn't remember seeing her last time we were here. This little old lady nurse looked somewhat more official. She had a couple of extra plastic card badges hanging from the lapel of her white medical coat which was exceptionally crisp and starched and it had navy blue stripes around the bottom edge of her sleeve. She almost appeared to be a military nurse or something.

Just have a seat here. Albert and I both sat in chairs along the wall of an examination room that she guided us to and the military nurse immediately started typing on a computer screen that sat on an arm like desk thing.

"How are you feeling today?" She looked at me and smiled with extremely dark red lipstick that was bleeding into the skin creases along her upper lip. Her hair was extremely straight and red; parted in the middle and chopped off into a rigid bob hairdo.

"Fine." I'm staring at her. I'm trying to figure out who she is still. I'm trying to figure out exactly what her role is because for some reason I can tell that she's not a typical nurse in the examination room. I'd be surprised if she actually works in this office every day. I think they brought her in special. She knows something. She's up to something. I don't know what it is but I know there's something going on.

"The doctor will be right in." She nodded politely, smiled and left the examination room.

"Interesting." I'm quiet as I nod my head in return.

"What?" Again with the what. Albert just doesn't get it.

Within less than one minute the door swung open and Dr. Alright was back in front of us once more. "How are we doing today?" He's pleasant but he's serious.

"Hello again." I'm smiling at him.

"Hello." Albert, the king of the one word sentences speaks.

Just behind the doctor, strolling right through the door as well is the military nurse and a very large man nurse. And suddenly I feel the hairs on the back of my neck stand up. I know the 'something's there' is finally here. And I now realize that the military nurse probably specializes in psychology. She's probably the one they always call when they're about to pummel you with horrific and horrible news about all of the 'something's theres' that secretly invade people's lives. She probably talks to us patients about coping, counseling, good nutrition and maybe even yoga. And the very large man nurse is obviously there for protection for the doctor, the military nurse, myself, and any other people that potentially are at risk if I or Albert are suddenly implosive human beings that want nothing more than to harm everybody around us because you just told us that I'm sick. Does the very large man nurse come to all of these appointments? Or did I cause his very presence as I stood over and behind my primary doctor's desk with my hands on my hips and demanded that he tell me what the 'something's there' is? Did my primary care doctor say something to them? Or did he put something in my chart? Is that why the girl at the front desk lost her smile? Is there a red flashing light that comes up when you open a patient's chart on the computer, which indicates that the patient is a potential hazard to the medical office's wellbeing? Am I considered a risk now? Or did the girl at the reception desk see the diagnosis?

"I haven't received the entire results from the biopsy yet."

What? Why? It's been two days like you said!!! Where are the results? I'm waiting here! I've done everything all of you have suggested already. I've made and kept all of the appointments. I've politely waited and I haven't bothered anybody with a bunch of phone calls or ridiculous questions. I think I've been a pretty good patient thus far and I don't deserve to be kept waiting. And I wasn't really angry or anything when I was asking my primary care doctor what the 'something's there' was; I just wanted to know what the 'something's there' is! There's just been a big misunderstanding about that. Why are you doing this to me? I'll bet if the patient was one of your family members you'd have gotten the results the very day they poked the long metal tube with the biting beak into their back!

"Okay." I shrug my shoulders and attempt to quiet my thoughts enough that I can pay attention to the doctor.

"I have received the initial report only."

"Well what does the initial report say?" The report comes in pieces? That's interesting. What would that look like? Sort of like an order being placed at a restaurant maybe? The waiter knows you're ordering an entire meal and initially you just order a drink and an appetizer. But the meal isn't complete until you order the actual meal, I suppose. Are we waiting for the meal? Does the report only tell us what the drink and appetizer is? Or are we waiting for the dessert part of the order!? Are we waiting for a giant slice of warm apple pie with a melting scoop of vanilla ice cream on top?!

Warm. Oh shit. That did it. It's getting hot in here again! I can feel it coming and it's starting in the center of my very core. I immediately start rubbing the back of my neck with one hand and fanning myself with the other.

"Are you okay?" The military nurse is speaking. She's just staring at me.

"I'm fine. Just a bit warm is all." I'm closing my eyes as I continue to try and make the air move just a teensy bit with my fanning hand in front of my face.

"Do you need some water?" A male voice asked me that question and I'm thinking it was the very large man nurse because I don't think I've heard the voice prior to this moment.

Why is it so dark in here all of the sudden? Did they just dim the lights or something? And it smells. It smells like sweet rotten dirt or something. I just need to take a breath, that's all. I lean my head back and literally gulped a huge breath of air, that I longingly wanted to be the cold crisp air that we ran through in the parking lot when we entered the building. But it wasn't. The air was hot and dripping with stale stank dew. In horror I opened my eyes and realized I was stuck in the hand dug well along the edge of the Canterbury property again. OH, NO! Please not again! Why does this keep happening to me?!

"No. I'm fine." I don't need water. I need air! There's water all around me. It's dripping down the walls of the well and my skin is completely drenched in the succulence of its rotten stench. My hair is twisting and tangling in the roots that are stabbing through the sides of the well as I continue to slip further and further into it. I can't grab hold of any of the sticks and branches, because they too are rotten and as quickly as I grab hold of them they smear across my palms as nothing more than greasy root carcasses. I can hear the water dripping into the huge pool at the very bottom of the well and I can hear something splashing about. What the hell is at the bottom of this freaking well?!

"I'm hoping to have the final results by tomorrow afternoon."

Why doesn't he just say what he knows? Why is he delaying the telling me of what he already knows? What was the drink and appetizer order? Who the hell is this guy? Why is he doing this to me? And what is that splashing?? What is the freaking splashing at the bottom of this well? And the more I struggle to keep myself from falling the more my panicking causes the sides of the well to begin to cave. They are caving in and they are covering my body with thick hot mud that smells like manure.

The closer I'm getting to the pool at the bottom of the well, the more intense the splashing is becoming! And I'm completely positive that the splashing must be an entire swarm of rats! And they're not the white rats that frolic through the tiny mazes in the science lab at school chasing after a small orange slice of cheese. These freaking rats are city rats. These rats are the size of small dogs! These rats didn't just innocently fall into the old abandoned hand dug well along the edge of the Canterbury property. These rats dove into the well because they smelled the rotting bodies of tiny animals that actually HAD innocently fallen into the well and drowned.

"Do we come back tomorrow then?" I can barely speak! I'm swimming in thick rotten mud now. The sides of the well are practically gone. The mud has slowly turned from a clay like substance to quick sand. The more I'm struggling the more the mud is covering me and diminishing any hope I have of finding just one gulp of clean cold crisp air.

"I will call you with that information or I will have the nurse call you."

"Okay." My voice sounds muffled and immersed within my mind as I fall and slither through what remains of the sides of the old hand dug well. The splashing is so intense now that I know it is just beneath me. The swarm of rats is gnashing and snarling as they leap through the pool and try to reach the sweet flesh along the underside of my feet. There's no light at all, as I continue to slip and slide further towards the horrific splashing! I can't see anything at all and I'm completely certain that I am about to suffocate within the smearing collapsing walls of the Canterbury well! I just need to breathe! I need to find a pocket of cold crisp air within the stench filled muck and mud that is covering my entire body! Somebody help me! I need to find the air and breathe! Do something, please! Somebody help me! PLEASE!!!

"At this point with the initial findings of the biopsy, I'm comfortable saying it's cancer."

And just like that it was out.

Chapter 18

I don't remember how I got out of the well along the edge of the Canterbury property. I don't remember anybody reaching in and grabbing ahold of my flailing arms and hoisting me up and out of the thick dank dark mud. Perhaps it was the large male nurse. Perhaps he was there to pull me up and out of the well before my body collapsed and I completely suffocated or drowned amongst the horrific splashing of the city rats. Perhaps he was the one that heard me screaming for help. A total and complete stranger heard me calling and screaming for somebody to do something or anything at all and just help me to find the air and breathe before my body completely died!

And as soon as I gulped in the air and began to recover from the horror within the well, I immediately felt like I was going to die again. And I remember falling forward.

"I need to call my mother." I'm staring straight out the windshield as we drive back to the off season rental cottage.

"Yeah." Albert's saying nothing for the most part. Neither one of us has words right now.

We're both in shock. We both were sure that it was a waste of time. We both were sure that we were going to be driving home and bitching about the wasted money for wasted medical appointments and wasted tests that freaking hurt!

"Hi Mom."

"Hi honey. What did they say?" She's nervous. I can hear her blowing smoke while she's waiting for me to answer the question. My mother's always smoked. I remember being five years old and getting yelled at to get out of the living room, because she was in there smoking and she didn't want us kids around it. In fact my entire family has always smoked. I don't know if I can actually think of an Uncle that doesn't smoke. Back in the early days of my life it was almost as if the entire world smoked and they just didn't worry about it back then. Nobody talked about cancer back then.

I remember the first time I smoked. I was only about ten years old. We, the family, were staying at my Uncle's camp on a tiny little lake way upstate Maine. We were there for an entire week. My cousins came to join us on one of the weekends and all of us kids set out exploring through the woods while the adults were cooking dinner on a barrel shaped barbeque grill in the backyard. As we trudged through the forest we stumbled upon an old Volkswagen van that was abandoned in the middle of the woods. We immediately busted into it which really only amounted to opening the side door and going inside. We played around for a while and realized that the old van had probably been used years ago as a quiet little get away for somebody that just wanted to relax along the side of the lake. There were dusty old blankets, a few shirts, and a few empty cans of beans and beer. In the tiny, rusty, pull-out ashtray on the dashboard we found some half smoked cigarettes and in the glove box we found a couple of books of matches. That was it! We smoked!

Years later when my parent's divorced and I felt a bit rebellious I decided that smoking was the perfect way to take control of my life. It was a way that I could feel like I fit in with the literally hundreds of other kids that smoked. It was a way that I could feel like an adult. Like I was grown up and in charge of the things around me. Like the way all of my Uncles felt as they sat around the Thanksgiving Day table smoking and laughing with their brothers, wives and children. I was a member of the 'in charge' club and it was no big deal. And back then it really was no big deal.

The first job I ever had when I was in High School was working at a local Bradlees store. I was a Housewares associate. I worked just a few shifts a week and most often got dropped off by my mother and driven home by a friend or boyfriend because I was still too young to have a driver's license. Well, at the very back of the store on the second level was the employee break room. That break room was nothing but a thick blanket of smoke. Every single person that worked at the store smoked. When you walked into the room, you quite literally couldn't see the people at the far end of the room.

When I finally moved out of my mother's house and into my own apartment, I had a job as a bartender. I smoked. I smoked a lot. Everybody did. The bar was the hottest spot in the Old Port, of Portland Maine. There was a dancefloor and lots of room to meet people and misbehave. It was a party every night! And everybody smoked. The entire club was filled with a giant cloud of tobacco smoke. And as the end of our shifts, my friends and I would go out for breakfast and we would eat, drink coffee, and smoke until six o'clock in the morning. That's what everybody did.

Years would go by before I finally stopped smoking. Of course I stopped a number of times over the years and when I took those breaks from smoking I had stopped for a number of years at a time. But nonetheless I used to smoke.

And it's odd to me that all of this pops into my head as I listen to my nervous mother blowing smoke throughout whatever room she is sitting in while she nervously asks me what the surgeon said. And I worry that perhaps... just perhaps...I did this to myself.

"Well, he doesn't have the final results of the biopsy just yet."

"What??!!" She's as frustrated as I was when the surgeon first said that.

"He hopes to have everything by tomorrow afternoon and then he'll call me."

"Okay. But why doesn't he have that now? It doesn't take that long! If it were his kid going through this he'd have had the results a freaking hour after they did the biopsy!" My mother is literally screaming. She was a nurse for years. She knows and she's screaming exactly what I was already thinking!

"Well he did have some findings."

"Okay."

"He is confident that it is cancer, Mom."

She says nothing. I can hear the smoke as it continues to blow through the room.

"He believes it is Mesothelioma because of the rare presentation. The tumors are in the pleura lining around the right lung. They are not in the lung itself."

I can hear my mother crying now.

"Mom! It's going to be okay. I'm going to be fine, stop worrying!"

She's struggling for her breath and it's killing me that I'm having this conversation with her over the telephone. I wish we lived closer to each other. I wished she were with me right now. I wish I could hug her while I tell her that I have cancer. I wish that she would stop the crying right now and just tell me that everything is going to be just fine. But how can she? How can she breathe right now as she blows out smoke and listens to her daughter tell her that she has cancer?

"It might not be Mesothelioma though! We will know tomorrow. The surgeon told me as we were leaving that I will get a call tomorrow, hopefully before noon. He said that if it were anything really serious he would be the one to call me directly. If not him then he will have one of the nurses in the office call me with the details about the final findings."

There's a long pause of silence and I know that the silence exists because my mother has set the phone away from her mouth as she struggles to compose herself. I know that my mother is sitting there, alone in her den, with the volume on the television turned way down so she can be sure that she doesn't miss a single syllable of the conversation. And I'm positive that as she hears the news she is picturing me a child. I'm positive she is picturing me running across the back lawn with my long blonde hair blowing in the breeze behind me. Either that or she is picturing me sliding down the big hill that ran along the border of our house in Westbrook, Maine just before I quite literally flipped the entire sled upside down and landed directly on my head!

"I have to call you later." She can barely speak and just hearing her voice and her struggle with such agony to even gather enough breath to produce those six short words breaks my heart.

"Mom. I'm going to be okay."

"I love you babe." And then she hung up.

The giant big man car pulled into the driveway in front of the tiny off season rental cottage as I looked at Albert. Tears were running down my face just as they had when I emerged from within the darkness of the Canterbury well back at the surgeon's office. It was at that very moment that I recalled; Albert was the one that saved me. Albert was the one that had heard my cries and had reached into the well as far as his body would allow. Quietly and softly my husband had saved me from drowning in the dark dank putrid mud filled with horrific bacteria. And when the surgeon spoke those words and my body fell forward Albert moved in closer and rested my tears upon his shoulder.

"You okay?" He's looking at me with an expression full of nothing, which actually speaks volumes. My husband is worried.

"I'll be okay." I smiled at him. "That was a horrible telephone call."

Chapter 19

What do you do when you hear that you have cancer? How do you settle? How do you stop thinking and wondering what is going to happen next? It's like the very second that the C-word is introduced as new vocabulary for defining your life, your mind comes to a screeching halt. The world continues to spin on its tilted axis, cars still speed by the house that you live in, the phone continues to ring, and the birds continue to fly on waves of an invisible wind that can either relieve you when it's too hot or knock you over as you struggle to stand tall within the fiercest of storms. Thoughts become frozen as if they are floating above our bodies and watching life as it continues to travel along paths, down streets, through forests and over vast acreages of land. The trick is to bring it all back together I think.

After we ate our take-out dinner of Chinese food and sat on the ugly couches in the ugly living room of the tiny off season rental cottage to watch television, I just couldn't sit still. I needed answers. Of course I found myself immediately turning to the internet. I grabbed the laptop and began slap-tapping the hell out of the keyboard.

"What are you doing?" Albert had turned the news on, which seemed to be screaming throughout the cottage.

"Researching. Gathering information. Trying to find answers to the burning questions within my frozen brain."

"Researching what?"

"Mesothelioma."

He stops watching the television and is just staring at me now. "You really think that's a good idea?"

"Well, what would you do?" I'm glaring at him now. Immediately he senses that I'm in no mood to explain my actions to him and he returns to watching the news. As I surfed and browsed and read whatever information popped up on the laptop screen, I wondered to myself 'what the hell did people do years before the internet even existed?' Where were the answers back then? How did anybody cope with NOT getting immediate gratification when they needed answers to burning questions?

And then I thought to myself, 'I guess they didn't.' People that had been introduced to the C-word back then had no means to research. They didn't even have a shred of the information that we have now and right at our fingertips. They must have just continued to remain frozen as life continued pulsating around them.

Whatever questions popped into their heads throughout the day, in the middle of the night or in the wee hours of the morning must have just waited. Those thoughts would just gather and stand in the corner of the living room as more and more thoughts joined the party. The thoughts would just continue to multiply until there would be an entire crowd of pushing and impatient thoughts all clustered together as a large group of strangers. Soon the entire corner of the living room would be so full that the thoughts would start bumping into each other. Their elbows and hips would shove into the next thought as drinks slurped and spilled over the edges of their glasses and stained the light tan shag carpet. And the volume of noise in the living room would continue to grow and grow until nothing else could be heard except for the screaming questions that completely invaded the once quiet and empty corner of the living room. Eventually the thoughts would all be taken with the person to an appointment with an Oncologist. Then and only then the dozens and dozens of thoughts would be heard and hopefully some answers would be offered to the unlucky soul that was introduced to the C-word.

By the time the news was over my research had ended and I closed the laptop. Everything that I read and every question I entered offered me no good news. I had read quite enough and wanted nothing more to do with the Mesothelioma research project. Quietly I tiptoed away from the ugly living room and into the master bedroom. "I'm getting my pajamas on." It was a feeble excuse but nonetheless an excuse to get into the next room without a need to explain what I was really about to do. Albert was flipping through the few available channels as I shut the bedroom door.

I did do what I said I was going to do; I did get my pajamas on. And as soon as I got my pajamas on I laid down on the bed for just what I thought would be a few seconds. I just needed a few small tiny little seconds. Just a few seconds to think about the day.

Just a few seconds to be alone with myself. Just a few seconds to relax and float atop the horribly hard mattress, with pillows under my head and three heavy blankets around my shivering body. Just a few seconds to be within my own thoughts and to not have to talk to anybody. No questions, no tests, no researching, and no comments whatsoever. I just needed a simple moment of nothing and I thought if I just rested in the darkness by myself with nothing but my own mind, I could maybe start to breathe again.

The moment never came though.

Just as I laid down on the bed and curled into the blankets and pillows, I suddenly felt the air becoming more and more humid. The entire room seemed to become thick and the oxygen seemed to be sucked away from the very air that floated around my body; the very air that I relied on for life giving breath was being invaded by this horrific thick hot humid air. How is it at all possible that it can be so incredibly cold but at the same time impossible to find some crisp air to breathe because it is so incredibly thick, rancid and hot?! Oh, NO! Why is it getting so hot again?!

I found myself immediately throwing the blankets off of my body and flailing my arms out and away from my sides. I struggled to sit up in the bed and slice through the air with my arms hoping to cause the layers and layers of stench filled heat to lift off of my body and allow some oxygen to penetrate my lungs! What the hell is happening?! I wanted to yell out loud with all of my strength and fury but I couldn't find any air to breathe so I could scream! I was flipping and flopping back and forth across the top of the incredibly hard bed as I struggled and struggled to escape the thickness of the air that pressed down upon my body! As I rolled and flailed I suddenly and without warning found myself rolling right off of the edge of the horribly hard bed! I could still hear the television blasting from the ugly living room in the off season rental cottage. Undoubtedly Albert was perched along the edge of the sofa with the remote tightly clasped in his right hand.

As I felt myself falling over the edge of the bed I could hear the volume of the television beginning to echo and beat within my ear drums. It sounded the way the wind sounds when somebody rolls down a rear window in the car as you speed down the highway. The further and further I fell away from the bed the more the pulsating pressure within my ears grew. My head hurt! I felt as if my skull were about to implode as the horrific pressure continued to grow as I continued to fall! I thought to myself: 'How far away is the top of the bed from the floor?!' I kept expecting to slam into the cold carpet covered floor with a thud, but the end of my fall wasn't coming! My body just kept falling and falling deeper and deeper as the pressure within my ears grew and grew. The more that I fell the further and further away the television sounded. My arms continued to flail and my legs seemed to be kicking out in all directions as I twisted and flipped through an unending hole of complete darkness.

Where the hell have I gone?! Why can't I get out of this horrific nightmare? Why is this happening to my body and how am I going to find myself, when I don't even know where I am?! Within seconds I could no longer hear the television screaming from the living room where Albert continued to sit. I was becoming more and more lost and felt my body falling deeper and deeper through a never ending hole of immense pressure. I had completely lost control of myself as I just kept falling! I struggled to see any hint of light or shapes within the darkness but there was nothing there. Nothing but sensations of depth and thick hot air as I spun and spun through the deepest and blackest of holes. My thoughts were racing as my struggle continued. How can there be nothing?! How can I be struggling to grab hold of something and keep from falling any further, but there is nothing to grab hold of? How can I be struggling to keep my eyes open when there is completely nothing to focus on? Where have I fallen to and how am I going to escape this hell?! I was screaming! I was screaming and flailing as my body exploded into a full state of panic! Why is this happening to me?!

The air was all around me and it was hot as I spun and flapped against the horrific breeze as my body just kept falling. Is this what happens to us? Am I dying as I'm falling deeper and deeper into the darker and darker air that has not even a shred of oxygen for me to continue to breathe? As my mind began to wonder and try to form some sort of reason, I could feel myself begin to slow down. I was still falling but everything began to move in slow motion. My world became completely surreal as I felt the hotness of the air begin to slide over my skin. The hot humid air was now a thick layer of mud that seemed to be covering my skin like a thick layer of chocolate frosting on a cake. My body was still struggling to flail and twist but I was quickly becoming encased and covered with a thick horrific layer of slime and mud. And the smell of the mud was overwhelming. I don't know what death smells like but I'm sure the smell of the mud that my body was entrapped within is exactly what it smells like. And the thick hot mud filled hole that smelled of rotten decay and bacteria infested filth overcame me. It overcame me and it took complete control of any and all of my efforts to have just that one quiet moment. And when I realized that I was completely and utterly hopeless as my being continued to fall and slide deeper and deeper into the succulence of putrid stench, I could do nothing within my feeble mind but continue to scream. I stopped flailing and I stopped spinning. I stopped fighting and I just let myself continue to slide deeper and deeper into the stench of mud that filled the deepest and darkest of all holes. The only thing I had left was one final effort to fill my lungs with one final breath of clean crisp air. With all of my effort and energy I gulped through the thickness of the putrid slime and I gasped and struggled to breathe! I needed to know! I needed to have the one question that was burning within my heart answered!

All of the other details on the internet were at my fingertips. I could punch in any question and have the details spill out right in front of me. No crowd standing in the corner of the living room bumping into each other and spilling drinks over the carpeting. No need to wait for the appointment with the Oncologist to ask the hundreds of questions that initially rolled through my mind. But there was that one tiny question that remained. That one question that the internet could find no answer to. And it needed to be asked. I needed to know. I needed to breathe so I could just ask that one tiny simple question!

I suddenly knew where I was. I knew where my body continued to fall and I wanted with all of my heart to keep it from continuing to happen! I don't know why I keep finding myself completely and utterly overwhelmed and back within the thick mud encased walls of that freaking hand dug well along the edge of the Canterbury property. And now I'm shaking my head back and forth with a vengeance as I struggle to regain my composure and pull myself up from the fall away from the bed but I had already fallen too far into the horrific bowels of that hand dug well! I could hear the thrashing and splashing of the swarm of rats again as they swam below me. They were getting closer and closer as I slid further and further towards them. They were so close to my body now that I could feel the thick slime of the pool beneath me lashing towards the skin on the bottom of my feet! The pool must be boiling because the heat from the splashing of slime that is reaching my skin feels like it is burning my flesh. The soles of my feet quickly turn into a layer of blisters as the boiling slime slaps my tender skin.

I needed to breathe! I needed air! As my body slid and slipped closer and closer to the swarming of the rats, I turned my head slightly to the right and tipped it back so I could make one final effort to find just a hint of crisp air. There had to be air because those freaking rats continued to breathe as they gnashed and chomped beneath my feat. I just knew there had to be a small pocket of air within the stench filled well and I needed to find it. I twisted and turned my head as my body slid through the last few feet of the hand dug well. And suddenly I felt it. I felt a sliver of cool dry air passing over my slime covered lips. I gulped and I gasped and heaved my body forward as the air passed through my mouth, down my throat and filled my lungs enough that I could scream with all of my might! I screamed as loud and horrifically as my body would allow. It was with all of my energy that I called out and cried towards the heavens. I needed to know. I needed to ask the one question that the internet could not give me an answer to!

"WHYYYYYY??!!!"

My scream seemed to shake the very walls within the tiny cabin as I suddenly slid to the very bottom of the horrific and putrid hand dug Canterbury well. I needed help! I could not get myself up and out of the well and I just knew within my very soul that this was exactly how I would die. The mud was completely covering every inch of my body. My hair was a long thick mane of slime and dirt. My eyes were shut and my lips were sealed. The rats crawled over and round my ankles as my feet slid into the boiling pit of decay and filth that they swam through. Quietly, I stopped the struggle, I hung my head and I just gave up.

"Are you okay?"

Albert quietly opened the door to the master bathroom, which I had somehow crawled into and crumpled myself into a ball on the floor just in front of the tub. There was a tiny little bathroom rug and I had tucked myself onto it. I was completely shivering. I was completely frozen as I laid there in a little ball of flesh on the tiny bathroom carpet. And I was crying. I was shivering and I was crying. My husband leaned down and gently scooped me up and into his arms. I struggled to stand and I leaned with every ounce of my weight into my husband's arms as I just continued to cry and shiver. He pulled me up and out of that well once again and I just crumbled into his arms.

I don't know how long I stood there in my husband's arms and cried. I cried so long and so hard that I quite literally ran out of breath. I couldn't talk. I was barely breathing even as my body heaved and choked with the deepest and most guttural cries of my entire life. It was at that very moment that I quite literally felt like nothing. I felt as if I was not a body. I had no brain. I had no mouth. I had no breath. I was nothing but a bundle of complete and utterly raw emotions. And I could not stop crying.

Albert just hugged me. He knew. He knew I needed him. And he came and he found me. And he lifted me up and out of that horrific well once again and then he hugged me. I knew it was because of his loving arms that I was able to stand up at all, as I sobbed in the tiny master bathroom in the off season rental cottage.

He kept telling me it was going to be okay. He kept rubbing my back as he held me up and calmed me down. He kept saving me as I kept falling over and over again. Logically I reasoned with myself and told myself that this whole C-word thing was stupid and it would absolutely not be the end of me. Logically I knew that I was going to be okay. Yet still I found myself slipping over and over again and deeper and deeper within the horrific well that lurked along the edge of that property. I didn't know how to make it stop happening.

Finally I stopped crying and leaned back to look into my husband's eyes. I knew he didn't have the answer to that one question that burned. There's no reason to even ask that question of him because I already know he won't have the answer. As I stared at him I thought about our life together. I thought about our five beautiful children and how lucky we were to have each of them in our lives. Through the years we had made it all work. We had provided it all one way or another and we had done a pretty good job as husband and wife. I was so proud of what we had accomplished together and I was so thankful to have done it with my husband at my side.

"It's going to be okay." He was staring at me and I could tell that he was choking on tears.

I just stared at him. There was only one comment that I could make. I wasn't going to say, 'I know…it's going to be okay. I'll be fine,' because that wasn't what overcame me at that moment. I wasn't thinking of my own survival. I wasn't thinking of the news that the doctor shared with us. I wasn't thinking of the hundreds of details that I'd just read on the internet before slipping back into the stench filled well. The only thing I was thinking and needed to express to my husband was wrapped within a thick blanket of incredible and overwhelming guilt.

How could I have done this to him? What had I done to myself to cause the 'something's there' to invade our lives? How could I have so carelessly created such hardship for my husband of nearly thirty years and our five beautiful children?!

I spoke only two words. There were only two words worth speaking as far as I was concerned. Two words that would tell him how much I never wanted to ever do anything that would cause him any pain whatsoever. Two words that would tell him that I never would intentionally do anything that would cause pain for our five beautiful children. The children that we had created together and the children that either one of us would die for without hesitation. Two words that would tell him that as many times as I tell him he's in trouble with me and as many times as I make fun of him within my own mind, he truly is the first one that I think about with every waking day. And as I stared directly into my husband's eyes I finally said it. I said it because it was what overwhelmed me even more than that one particular question that the internet couldn't find an answer for. It overwhelmed me to the point that I could not keep myself from falling into the horrific dark stench of the Canterbury well. It overwhelmed me to the point that I couldn't stop worrying and thinking about what my husband would now be facing within the emptiness of our new home in Laconia, New Hampshire. It overwhelmed me to the point that I couldn't stop thinking that our five beautiful children do not deserve what may be coming. Because of me. So I said it. I looked deeply into my husband's eyes and I told him exactly how I felt. I told him what he deserved to hear because he didn't deserve what was now happening to us and our children.

"I'm sorry."

Chapter 20

"Do you work today?" Albert's just now stumbled through the living room. I've been up for three hours now and can think of nothing other than my telephone ringing.

"Unfortunately."

"What do you mean?"

"I mean I close tonight. I go in at two o'clock. And I mean I don't want to. I can't stop worrying about that freaking phone call. I don't want to play 'leader' to a bunch of people that truly deserve a true leader when I can't focus on being the person I was hired to be because I am too wrapped up in myself right now and whether or not I am going to be alive in another year!" I'm beginning to become irritated with Albert for no reason whatsoever and he better not for the love of God tell me it's going to be okay. I swear to God if he says that to me when I'm sitting here on my fourth cup of coffee freaking out and just waiting…because that's ALL I've been able to do now for I don't even know how many days I'll kill him! I will freaking tackle him right to the floor and pound on his ass! I swear to God he better not say it!

"It'll be okay."

I'm glaring at him like an angry bull.

"What?" He's stuck. He has absolutely no idea. How can somebody be that oblivious?

"I'm going to take a shower." Quickly I stand up and stomp through the living room, into the bedroom and into the master bathroom. And I know I'm stomping out of the room right now for two different reasons: One, because I need to take my mind off the 'waiting.' Two, because if I remain within reach of Albert right now his life will truly be in danger.

"What'd I do?" He's calling after me and I imagine he's still standing there in the kitchen with his arms flailing out at his sides.

The minute I get into the shower I feel better. The water is so warm and inviting and somehow I feel like it's going to be okay. How can it not be okay? This is not my life! I am not one of those people that gets sick! I'm so healthy! This doesn't make sense to me. I know I smoked years ago but so did the rest of the entire freaking world. And even if I hadn't smoked for all of those years, I in effect would have been smoking anyway because the smoke was everywhere! You couldn't avoid it. It was in every restaurant, break room, home, the bars, the nightclubs, and for Christ's sake you could even smoke in hospitals back then! How can it be that I am one of the ones that has been singled out? I must have done something else to myself! It can't have been the smoking!

Mesothelioma; I looked it up. It is caused by asbestos exposure. It's not caused by smoking! But, when the hell did that freaking asbestos shit happen to me? Was it one of the houses that we bought and rehabbed? Is that where it came from? Was it one of the twenty houses that Albert and I have purchased over the past thirty years? The houses that we purchased as investments for our family? The houses that Albert slaved away in for weeks, ripping out walls, floors, insulation, plumbing, and electrical? Only to put it all back together and sell it within just a few short months for our family's well-being and financial security. Or was it not one of the investment properties and it was one of the houses that we actually lived in and I raised our children in? Was it the first house we ever bought? Did I touch something I wasn't supposed to in the basement? Was there a thick piece of plaster looking tape hanging off a heating pipe and it was flapping in the breeze right in front of my face as I made my way to the washing machine and I reached up and simply tore it off the pipe? Were there teeny little microscopic pieces of asbestos dust that flew into the air and I just happened to inhale as the dust particles flew and the particles lodged inside of my right lung? Have they been growing and developing into tumors for the past twenty five years? Is that what happened to me?

And when all of these thoughts were raging through my brain, I kept my face pointing directly into the shower stream. My eyes were clamped shut and I was constantly spitting water out of my mouth as I brushed the stream off my cheeks. I loved the feeling of the water running over my face at that moment. It was soothing. I was almost relaxing even though my thoughts just could not stop.

And then it started again. It started again like the streaming of the water had washed away a thick mask of creamy white makeup and once again my emotions were revealed. And the dripping of the thick white makeup was practically chocking me and blocking the air, which couldn't break through the wave of paste that covered gasping mouth. But the good thing about the water running over my face was that nobody would ever be able to tell that I was crying again. With the water running into and out of my mouth and the sputtering of the thick white paste, it was also completely impossible to scream. I couldn't help but want to keep my emotional instability a secret. Nobody needs to know that I can't stop this. My children do not even know what is going on yet. They know I'm waiting for biopsy results. They know about everything up until yesterday afternoon. I can't see making all of the calls until we know exactly what the hell is freaking going on! Up until now they've all been kept informed of every single detail and every time I talk to every single one of them, they all keep saying the same thing to me: "It's going to be okay, Mom. You'll be fine." None of them think that anything can ever happen to their mother. They don't believe it. They won't believe it. And I can't tell them right now. I can't even say the word. How can I? How can I even let that word slip between my lips? I can't do it! I don't know what to do! It simply cannot be that I have Mesothelioma! How on earth am I going to tell my five beautiful young adult children that I've just been handed a death sentence?

I'm completely overwhelmed! I can't even freaking breathe! I don't know what to do but I need to get away from this! My instinct is to just run. Run as fast and as furiously as I can away from the danger and into an area that will protect me from the danger that's chasing me. The danger is chasing me as if I'm running through a dark forest that the sunlight can't ever permeate. The trees are tall and the branches are completely covered with millions and millions of dark green leaves. And the millions of leaves on the millions of branches are high in the air and they create a canopy over the entire forest. The forest floor is nothing but a thick spikey blanket of pine needles that I am forced to run over with nothing but naked feet. And there is no life in the forest. There are no animals frolicking through the woods. There are no flowers, no insects, and there is no breeze. Just the darkness and the huge trees. And I'm just running! I'm running fast and furiously straight ahead of where I stood silently just moments before. And behind me as I scramble and twist and turn my body through the thick sharp branches, I can hear something coming. It's coming up behind me and it's not going to stop until it catches me. It's running after me! There are huge heavy beating footsteps coming up behind me and they are faster than my feet ever thought of being. And I'm trying and I'm trying to pick up my pace but I keep getting caught between branch after branch of the huge and horrifyingly dark trees. And I can't even scream anymore. I only have the energy to run and run as fast as I can. And I'm so terrified that I'm actually vomiting in the back of my throat. I'm vomiting and I'm running and the footsteps are nearly upon me now! I swear to Christ I can feel the breath of the thing that's chasing me on the very back of my neck and I just know that it's reaching out for me! And it's bigger and it's more powerful than I could have ever imagined and I don't know how I'm going to get away from the horrific and horrible gripping clamp that's about to be upon me!

"Are you okay?" There's more pounding. There's more pounding all around me and I struggle to open my eyes. What the hell else can possibly be happening to me now? I twist and turn and struggle to breath but all I can do it sputter and spit a mouthful of water.

"Honey, are you okay?"

Shit, that's Albert! How is it that he keeps catching me? Suddenly I manage to open my eyes and realize that I'm still okay. The water has run cold and I'm completely shivering as I stand in the tiny shower in the master bath.

"I'll be right out." Quickly I turn off the water and leap through the bathroom toward the thickest and the biggest towel that I have folded atop the tiny shelf that balances over the back of the toilet bowl. I can't dry off quick enough to rid my body of the horrific cold that is permeating through my skin and into the depths of my bone. Quickly I scoot into the bedroom and dress in the warmest sweatpants and fleece shirt from L.L. Bean that I could find in the freaking suitcase that I'm still living out of. When I finally emerged into the living room Albert asked me the same question, again.

"You okay?"

"Yeah. Just want the phone to ring. And I know the second

I hear the voice I'll know if it's bad or good news. Because if it's the surgeon...it'll be more serious. That's what he said. He said he would be the one to call if it was Mesothelioma." I plop onto the couch and begin watching the news with Albert. My hair is dripping wet as I pull the ridiculous afghan of brilliant coral and pea green towards me. And I can't help but wonder about the choice of the yarn colors; the person that made this must have just used up leftover skeins of yarn. Nobody would intentionally put coral and pea green together.

"What time is he calling?"

"As soon as he gets the rest of the report. Whatever time that means! Probably freaking tomorrow." The second the words came out of my mouth my phone began to ring-sing and I immediately snatched it up from the ugly homemade coffee table. I snatched it up with the reflex of a major league baseball pitcher as he snaps a line drive hit from the air and into the quick and meticulously worn glove on his left hand. "Oh shit! It's the doctor's office number!"

This is it! This is the call that I'm waiting for and the news that will tell me if I have six months to live or not! And the 'NOT' part of the information will be the good news. That's the news I'm hoping to hear from whoever at the surgeon's office is calling me right now. I'm shaking! I'm shaking so hard I can barely swipe the front of my phone to pick up the freaking call! I want to take the call but I don't want to take the call. I don't have any choice but face the fact that I am picking up a call from a surgeon or merely a person in his office that I've never even met and I don't even know, and that is the person that is going to tell me if I am going to die in less than a year. Why is this okay? Who are these people anyway? Why should I receive this kind of information from somebody that doesn't even know me? That surgeon doesn't know that I've been married for thirty years to a wonderful man. He doesn't know what my husband and I have survived already together and he probably doesn't even want to. He doesn't know that our first born child terrified us because his heart stopped beating two weeks prior to his due date and I had to be rushed into the hospital from the OBGYN's office. He doesn't know that my second oldest son is the most sensitive and caring person in the world, even though he has challenges. He doesn't know that my oldest daughter was the first wish I had that ever came true; it came true because SHE was born. He doesn't know that my two youngest, the identical twin girls, are the reason that people play the lottery every single week! How is the responsibility of telling me and my family whether or not we are about to be sucked into the vortex of a monstrous tornado of death bestowed upon a man that I don't know, just met, don't even know his first name, and have shared nothing about my love and my life with whatsoever?! But maybe it's not him! Maybe it's not the surgeon at all! Maybe it's the nurse that was so nice the first time we went to the surgeon's office. Maybe it's the military nurse!

"Hello." My voice is shaking as much as my hands are right now.

"This is Dr. Alright."

"Oh, no." Shit, it's the surgeon. Oh my God, it's the surgeon. Why did it have to be the surgeon? My stomach is burning. My heart is sinking. The room is suddenly so dark. The lights are dimming at an incredible rate and my internal body temperature is rising. My body temperature is rapidly rising and must be well over one-hundred degrees. Within the second that it took for my brain to compute that it was the actual surgeon on the other end of the telephone I have become immersed in nothing but blackness, my heart is no longer beating and I am completely and utterly still. I wasn't running through the darker than dark forest anymore. I wasn't falling through the thick dank mud inside the Canterbury well again. I was just sinking. I was sinking and sinking within my very skin as the utter core of my soul just collapsed with a deep and guttural sigh.

"I wanted to call you because we received the final results for the biopsy just now."

I can't even respond. A single tear is already running down my left cheek. My heart feels as if it is breaking. It's breaking for my children. It's breaking for my husband. It's breaking for my mother. I can't focus. I'm not breathing and I'm completely and utterly numb. I can't speak. That one single burning question is all that my being is about right now and I can think of nothing else but 'WHY? Why God is this happening to me?' How is it that my life has been ripped out from underneath me so suddenly and with no warning whatsoever?! What did I do? What shouldn't I have done? How did I do this to myself and what do I have to do to just make it all go away and we can all pretend that it never even happened in the first place!

'PLEASE, God just help me now!!!'

It's so quiet. Is he waiting for me to say something? I can't speak. I'm just silent as I wait to hear the surgeon's deep raspy voice say those words. The words that will tell me what is going to happen in my life and how long I have to possibly keep living or not. He needs to talk. He needs to just get it over with and tell me what has been delivered to me and my family.

He's breathing. I can hear him breathing into the phone and I hear him shuffling papers. Albert is sitting across the living room from me and he's just staring. He is waiting for a sign. A sign from me that the words being spoken on the other end of the phone are good. A sign that will tell him whether or not he needs to leap across the room and catch me from falling to my death at the bottom of the stench filled Canterbury well, again.

"Okay." It's all I can muster. It's the only thing I can get out of my mouth; just a short and simple acknowledgement that the phone connection is good and I can hear the words he's speaking.

But I already know the answer. He told me that he would be the one to call me if it in fact turns out to be Mesothelioma. He said that if it were anything other than that he would have one of the nurses in his office call and give me the news. I already know what it is. I already know that I in fact will probably be dead in just six months. How am I going to tell my children that I'm going to die? How am I going to call my mother and tell her that I won't make it to my next birthday? I won't have to tell Albert anything. He will know the second my expression reacts to the words from the surgeon.

Quietly I hung my head and I just breathed. The weight of my entire world pressed down upon the back of my shoulders. I braced myself. I braced myself with all of my thoughts and I listened for the words that the surgeon was about to speak.

There was no sound. No sound whatsoever. What is he doing? Why won't he speak? Then I suddenly heard him breathe deeply as he formulated just one simple sentence.

"It's not mesothelioma."

Chapter 21

"I don't have mesothelioma!" I'm shaking even more now as I scream the words to Albert. He's been sitting on the couch and he's been struggling to understand what the surgeon has reported to me. He only heard half of the conversation. He's been hanging over the very front edge of the couch and he's been straining and struggling to understand what exactly I've been hearing from the surgeon. And now that I've hung up all I can do is scream! "I'm not going to die! I don't have it!"

"What did he say?" Albert's standing up on the other side of the living room now with his mouth hanging open and his arms out to his side. He's smiling and he doesn't even know why.

"I don't have it!"

"Okay!"

"He said the final results are in and I do not have Mesothelioma. What a relief!" I can't stop smiling! I can't stop spinning from the news. I am going to be okay. I will get through whatever is thrown at me. This will not be the end of me. And SHAME on myself and shame on those that left me thinking for even a second that it was all going to be over in just a few short months! Who are they anyway? They are not me! They do not know me! And how dare they presume for even a moment that they would be giving ME that kind of news! How dare they believe that they are going to tell ME what is going to be. They DO NOT KNOW ME!

"Oh GOD! Thank you GOD!" Albert's literally falling. He's falling and he's completely lost his balance as his entire body collapses into the hideous couch in the off season rental cottage.

We laughed out loud, rubbed our heads, hugged, and breathed for at least five minutes before the next question came.

"What else did he say?" Albert's still smiling as he sits back down on the hideous blue couch. He's leaning forward on his knees and he has his face perched into his hands. He's excited and he wants all of the details. He wants a play by play recount of the entire conversation so he can revel in the words as I repeat them as if I were the surgeon speaking.

"Well, he said I have cancer." The words come out of my mouth and they feel like a fresh spring of cool crisp water that douses a smoldering fire at the very back of my horrifically dry throat.

"What?!" Albert's serious again.

"Yeah. I have cancer. But we knew that, right?" I'm staring at him. I'm watching his face as it completely freezes with no expression whatsoever and it dawns on me that perhaps Albert has just accidentally stepped foot into the rotten covering on the murky hand dug well along the edge of the Canterbury property.

Why is he so confused? The phone call that I just received was not to determine yes or no…it was to determine death or chance! Did he miss something? The surgeon had already explained to us during that last visit in his office when the military nurse and the great big man nurse stood there doing nothing, that he was comfortable sharing with us the diagnosis. He said he was comfortable saying it was cancer. He said he was waiting for the final results of the biopsy to determine the type. Well, now we know the type. And more importantly we know that it's not Mesothelioma! Did Albert hear none of that? Had Albert been standing there with a mind full of defiance the entire time? Had he heard the words but his mind was stuck in a state of 'I don't think so' this whole time? Has Albert been holding onto false hope that we were going to hit the Powerball?

We're not hitting the Powerball.

"So what else did he say?" Albert is so lost and confused and I wish I'd just put the call on speaker when it came through.

"He said it's Carcinoid Cancer and it's in the pleura lining of the right lung. He said I need to head to Boston. This is outside of what he typically deals with. He said this is extremely rare. And he said he would have a nurse contact me later today and they will help us get scheduled for a consultation with a Thoracic Surgeon in Boston as soon as they can get us in."

Albert's just staring straight ahead. He's not moving. He's not speaking.

"Are you okay?" I'm completely smiling! I feel like celebrating and I WISH I didn't have to go to work today. This feels like the sort of night that should be spent having dinner at a fancy restaurant, while I toss back a few margaritas with lots and lots of salt on the rim!

Still silence from Albert.

"What a relief!" I'm dancing. I'm dancing throughout the living room, into the kitchen to put away the coffee cups from this morning, back into the living room again, down the hall to pick up dirty towels in the bathroom, through the living room and kitchen to dump the towels into the washing machine and back into the living room again. And the whole time I'm smiling and I'm singing within my own mind as I thank the Lord for all that he has done and all that he continues to do for me.

Still nothing from Albert.

"Are you okay?" I'm stopping and I'm staring at Albert as I just continue to wait for him to speak. He's completely stuck and hasn't budged from his seat as I've danced through the cottage. This may be the only time I've ever seen my husband completely and one hundred percent speechless. He's not humming. He's not the king of the one word sentences. He's just frozen. I slowly stepped forward and stood directly in front of him with my hands on my hips.

"Albert! Are you okay?"

Quietly he looked up at me and then finally he spoke: "What the hell is Carcinoid Cancer?"

Chapter 22

I didn't even know how to answer Albert's question when he asked what the hell Carcinoid Cancer was; mainly because I don't know the answer to that question. I researched it immediately after I stopped jumping up and down and celebrating that I am not in fact going to be dead in just six short months.

Carcinoid Cancer is one of many types of cancers and it happens to be a slower growing cancer than some. (That is my good news) It is rare. It is a cancer that can metastasize but one that takes time to grow and spread. A type of cancer that can lurk in the shadows undetected for a period of years; masking many common ailments pretending to be that which it is not. It causes a person to continually trudge into the doctor's office complaining about the same discomfort over and over. It causes the doctor to do nothing more than write a handful of useless prescriptions, order a host of useless tests, and thereby determine that the patient is nothing more than 'getting old.' Exactly what I had assumed would be the outcome of my many appointments which followed the initial appointment I had at the Orthopedic Center because my shoulder hurt. I got lucky. I got lucky because they caught it. I got lucky because that one person at the Orthopedic Center who was looking for a torn rotator cuff suddenly saw something just outside of the viewing screen that was not in fact what he or she was looking for. And that one particular person scratched the side of his or her head and said, 'what the hell is that?' And then the call came to me. The call that said…'something's there.'

If that person that reviewed the MRI had not been on their game, I would have done nothing but scheduled an appointment for some useless strengthening physical therapy appointments because for an undetermined reason my shoulder hurt. And low and behold and according to the surgeon that is now sending me to Boston, the very cause of the pain in my shoulder is the tumors that are resting against major nerves that run underneath my armpit and between my ribcage and shoulder muscles. "The cause of your pain is right there," he said as he pointed to the computer screen.

"Good morning!" I walk through the store office and greet

my administrative assistant before passing her desk and heading to my office. She's always so pleasant. She's one of just a few that's already accepted me and figured out that I am truly a nice person regardless of the vicious rumors that the snake continues to spread.

The second I entered my tiny little office, threw my sweater across the back of my chair and put my lunch bag in the tiny little refrigerator in the corner, it hit me. It hit me like a tidal wave of emotions. Just a mere moment before it hit me I was relaxed and smiling. I was smiling and breathing as if I walked along a warm tropical shore wading in the ocean that I swear to God feels like bath water. And the air was so incredibly warm and comforting. And as I strolled along the very edge of the ocean I felt protected. I felt as if nothing can ever get any better than how I was feeling at that very moment. I knew everything was just going to be okay. I knew that all the comforts of the earth surrounded me and there would be nothing that could ever take it away from me.

But then out of nowhere it hit me. And when it hit, it hit hard and it knocked me clear off my feet. It must have been lurking out there in the very center of the ocean and some sort of underground earthquake or tremor must have given it life. Suddenly a giant tidal wave pummeled the very land that I stood firmly on just moments ago. And the tidal wave has no mercy. There's no thought behind the tidal wave. The tidal wave just lives to overwhelm. That is the only role of the tidal wave and unfortunately I was in the very path of its newly born life. And suddenly it overtook me. It scooped me up and off of my feet, as it carried me through thick mud and debris and across the land with a vicious whipping and swirling of my useless body. And I can't fight it. I can't fight against it because I just don't have the power that it would take to calm the brutal nature of a tidal wave. And even if I were to flail around and scream for help it simply would do no good. I am completely and utterly at the mercy of the force within an ocean.

I am helpless and all I can do now is just go along for the ride. And the ride intends to pull me out and into the middle of the vast and never ending ocean. Somewhere out in the middle of the ocean I am destined to just try and keep my head above the water. And it is at that very moment when I am floating in the middle of nowhere, that I will suddenly feel so incredibly small. Because it is then and only then that I suddenly realize, for perhaps the first time in my entire life, I have no true power on this earth. I do not have the power to fight against the tides of the ocean. I do not have the power to reverse what has been happening to me over the course of so many years now. I do not have the power to take it all away and make it so it never really happened at all. It has happened and I cannot change that.

So as I continue to float in the middle of the ocean, I suddenly realize that I cannot control my world. I cannot control what will happen to me. It will happen. It did happen. And in that instance when I realized that something had actually happened to me, I suddenly realized that I would never be able to control the waves. But in the same instance I realized that I still controlled what was deep within my very being. And it is because of that something that is deep within me that I am able to do anything at all! And it is within that short simple moment of realization that my mind suddenly shifted and I focused on that which I will be able to impact.

I cannot fight against the ocean. I cannot hold back the giant waves that toss me about like an empty soda bottle floating atop the currents. I cannot win a battle against the world. I absolutely cannot even for an instance make the ocean go away. It is here and it deep. And as deep as it is and as much as it swirls and twists and carries my body within its currents it still cannot control that which is within me!

Even though my body is twisting and twirling within the currents of the ocean, I can still swim!

Even though I have no idea where the currents are about to take me, I can still face the direction!

Even though my body may become tired and have those moments where it just wants to give up and just float, I can still scream at the top of my lungs and force myself to re-focus once again!

I can respond to the brutal force behind the ocean with all of my might! My body is one thing but my soul is quite another. My soul cannot be overcome. My soul is deeper than the very ocean that carries me now. My soul is not a tangible object so it is therefore completely untouchable. My soul is housed within my body and it contains my every desire, my motivation, my faith, my beliefs and my love. And my soul is strong. My soul will be what brings me through the currents. My soul is what learned to swim in the first place, when I was a mere five years old and stood shivering in the public swimming pool in Westbrook, Maine. And it is within that tiny little moment of realization as my body swirled atop the waves within the deepest part of the vast and powerful ocean that I suddenly began to swim.

"How did everything go with the surgeon?"

My administrative assistant is standing in my office. I have tears in my eyes as I try to form the words and tell her that I will be fine. The words that I know will be shared with the entire team once I speak them. The words that will need to show the team that although I am human and although I cannot control everything in this world, I still promise to be their leader and I will still put them first and foremost with all that we do to support the customers and the company that we work for. The words that will tell them all that I will be just fine.

She's still innocently staring at me and I wonder if she can tell that I am choking right now. I am choking as I struggle to keep my head above the water and maintain my role and form the words without a quivering voice. I am choking as I twist from side to side and with a slow and steady pace began to swim across the surface of the vast and powerful ocean. As I finally began to move through the cold frigid water, I managed to tell her: "I got good news from the surgeon just before I headed into work today."

"Oh?" She's smiling. She's genuinely happy for me.

My arms stretched high above my head and splashed water around my face, my feet were kicking as hard as I could kick them and I breathed in and out with the rhythm of my strokes.

"I have Carcinoid Cancer."

Chapter 23

When the hell did Albert forget how to drive? He's acting like a complete maniac as we maneuver around and through the confusing streets of Boston. Years ago when we first went for a family vacation to Puerto Rico he drove every single day. And none of us knew where we were going and of course none of us thought for even a moment that perhaps we should pack a GPS. Looking back, I think he did a phenomenal job of getting us around the island. This is especially true when one considers that NOBODY living in Puerto Rico can freaking drive! The driving on that island is completely treacherous! Nobody stops for red lights and they all speed and slam on their brakes for no reason whatsoever! The police cars always keep their blue lights on so when you see them anywhere near you, your instinct is to panic and pull over to the side of the road. AND there's about a million stray dogs that are forever strolling out and into the middle of the road! How did Albert get us through all of that but he can't seem to get us to my first appointment with a Thoracic Surgeon at Brigham and Women's Hospital in Boston, Massachusetts?

"Are you okay?" I'm staring at Albert with my mouth hanging open. He's perched himself at the very front edge of his seat, his face is a mere six inches from the windshield, he's twisting and turning his body constantly as he tries to watch every single car, pedestrian and the freaking blowing of the wind! And he keeps grunting! He's grunting like he's in pain as he twists and turns around in the car. It's like he doesn't fit into the vehicle and with every twist and turn he is in extreme pain as a portion of his body slams into the door, the arm of the chair, or the steering wheel. I don't think I've ever seen him in such a state of panic! What the hell is going on with him? I think he's going to have a heart attack just getting us to this freaking appointment!

"Just don't talk." He's completely losing it.

"Relax. We're almost there." And I guess I can understand some of his discomfort. I'm sure his body is probably sore; he's been spending every minute he can in between my doctor's appointments and melt-downs, getting our new home cleaned, carpeted, wood floored and painted. So I do 'get it' to some degree. Obviously he's stressing out. I'm just surprised at the level of his reaction, discomfort and frankly his whining.

"Do you want to drive?" Now he's getting angry.

"Yes." I'm staring at him.

I pause waiting for a response but he's immersed within his panic stricken mind. He says absolutely nothing.

"Do you think you can manage to pull over? I'll take over right now! It won't bother me at all!" Why the hell didn't I just drive? I should have taken over the car when we came to a screeching halt on the highway nearly an hour and a half ago. We were only ten miles from our exit at that time. And that's when all of the panic situated itself within Albert's mind. That's when he began shifting in his seat and rubbing his knees which I'm completely positive do not hurt! In fact his 'knee pain' is probably nothing more than sympathy pain. He has created a physical ailment within his own mind because he is overly stressed because of his wife's medical issue.

More silence.

I decided to stop harassing Albert. We are used to living in the middle of nowhere. Traffic for us is three cars at a stop sign. Any city compared to what we are used to driving through is scary; so I truly do understand what Albert is trying to manage through right now. I don't think he would be this big of a freak about the traffic though if his mind weren't already overwhelmed with the relocation and with me having cancer. That's all I'm saying. We'll get there. We are literally right down the road from where the hospital is supposed to be. He just needs to bring it down a few levels. And why the hell is he so nervous anyway? He's not the one facing whatever the hell it is that I'm facing! I'm the one that's got a freaking growth on the edge of my freaking lung! I'm the one dealing with the 'something's there'!!!

"It should be up here on the left." Albert's still grunting, even as he's speaking. He's leaning so far into the windshield he looks as if he's trying to smell the glass. And he's wrenching his head to the right as he's struggling to see to the very tippy top of a very tall building. What the hell is he looking for?

"I see it." I respond to Albert with a tone that seems to actually say, 'How can you miss it?' The building is completely huge with a giant sign above the door. There are actually a couple of different entrances. This building is like a whole block or something. And there are people everywhere! Most of them look like they work in the medical field. And they are walking everywhere! Down the street, across the intersections, into buildings, out of buildings, hailing taxi's, buying food and coffee, and they just appear to be constantly scattering and skittering back and forth in front of our car. Some of them are trying to eat the food they just bought so I imagine they are on a lunch break from work. Some of them look like it took longer than they had anticipated to even get into work for what must be the second shift for the hospital and now they can't scurry quickly enough through the intersections to get up to the seventh floor of the building where they clock in, work and man their station! Just watching the constant flow of pedestrians is mind blowing. Where do all of these people come from? How can they possibly keep track of what they need to do every single day when they come back into this world filled with traffic, huge buildings and so many other people darting around, in front of and past them? I could NEVER survive here! I'm completely positive that at the end of my first day on the job, were I to ever move to Boston which I totally would not even ever do but if I did, I wouldn't even be able to find my way back to my car. And what about all of the people that take a train to get here? Where the hell do they even go to find the train? I never even saw a train but I've heard that they for sure do really exist! And for that matter where are all the busses? There are busses aren't there? I've only seen like one bus and I swear to God it was a bus that belongs to some Country Western Singer, not a bus for normal people. I thought the big cities had busses that stopped on every street corner like every thirty minutes or so for all of the people that live in the city, have to get to work or school, but don't own a car to get there. Where are all the busses? There are definitely not enough busses in this city!

Oh my God. I'm completely lost!

"Where are we supposed to park?" Albert's voice is calming down. Now that he realizes we have arrived and we and the car are still in one piece, he's beginning to relax a bit. Even though my mind is completely scattered like the thousands of people that just don't seem to stop darting to and fro and everywhere in front of our car!

"They have valet parking."

"What?" His voice went up three octaves.

"That's what it says in the paperwork they sent me." I dig through my giant purse and pull out an envelope of neatly folded paperwork, a disc that has my scan on it, a copy of the biopsy report and instructions from the hospital we are just now arriving at. "First entrance, use valet parking service, it says so right here." I'm actually pointing to the paperwork like I expect Albert to stop driving and read it for himself. And I know he wants to because he completely doesn't believe that a hospital would have valet service because the only valet service we have EVER used in our entire lives was that one time at a country club when we dressed up in formal attire for a banquet/dinner/celebration thing and it was ten degrees below zero outside. We used the valet service that night so we wouldn't have to freeze to death walking the one-hundred yards to the car from the clubhouse and then back again.

"Okay then." He's shrugging as we pull in behind an entire row of turning vehicles that are also using the valet service for the hospital. As soon as it is our turn to get out of the car, collect a ticket, and get into the building it becomes even more obvious that we are the only two people within this entire city that have no clue whatsoever about where we are! Where are we going? How are we supposed to get there? And oh my GOD how on earth are we ever going to find our way back home when the day finally ends?!

"Where do we go?" Albert's voice sounds like a little girl's.

"I don't know. We need to find L2 off the elevators, turn right, walk to the third hall on the left past the gift shop, turn around the second corner to the right by the parking garage elevators, and look for the fourth office entrance on the left. And then we head toward the Thoracic Surgery area. And supposedly there's some sort of really long hallway that everybody travels on and they refer to it as a pike or something." I'm reading the instructions as we walk in circles within the huge front entrance atrium area of the building.

"Like the fish?"

"No. Like a turnpike."

"Do you need help?" Somebody that works here spotted us. For some reason we stood out to them.

127

Within mere minutes we are traveling along 'The Pike', heading in the correct direction. And mere moments after that we breathed a huge sigh of relief when we found ourselves actually sitting in the waiting room for the Thoracic Surgeon that I have an appointment with this morning. And this particular office is so calm and quiet and cool and they have actually put out free coffee, water, muffins and fruit Danish and pastry for the patients. For some reason Albert believes that he should be considered one of the patients because after all he did drive here and he immediately starts eating as much as he possibly can from the platter of free treats.

"Do you want some?" He's staring at me with wide open eyes, as he's beginning to scoff down Danish number two. "They're good."

"I'm all set." I'm staring back at him with a smirk on my face and Albert completely just doesn't get it. And I'm sure that the people that work here do not mind at all if the patient's guests/drivers/husbands have free food and drink; I'm sure they had that in mind when they made the decision to put out the platters every single day. But a very big part of me worries about that patient with obvious cancer and severe health issues, who will most assuredly enter the waiting room later today having just finished another round of chemo or radiation. And they've most assuredly been in this hospital for nearly twelve hours already and they've not had time to get a quick bite of anything to eat and they're going to plop themselves into a chair that sits directly next to what will most assuredly by that time be nothing more than an empty freaking platter of what used to be free food for them in case they really need it.

"Put some in your purse."

"What is wrong with you?" I'm angry now.

"What?"

"You can come in now." There's a pleasant nurse with a pleasing grin, beckoning me to come with her behind the door to the unknown.

"Thank God!" I quickly scurry through the door and can't help but be annoyed when I realize that Albert has managed to catch up with me and now is sitting with me in another waiting room which is really the examination room.

"How are you today?" The nurse is a normal person. She's not one of the cheerleaders. She's pleasant but she's talking like she's just another normal person in the world and she is genuinely nice but at the same time she's professional. She's not getting ready to lead an entire auditorium full of people in the chanting of the school's official song.

"I'm good."

"What brings you to us?"

"I had an incidental finding when I went to an Orthopedic Center for shoulder pain." The nice nurse is taking notes like a stenographer. "That led to an x-ray, which led to a C Scan, which led to a biopsy, which led to a diagnosis of Carcinoid Cancer."

"Okay." She's still typing. "Did you bring any discs?"

"Yes." I quickly begin digging through my purse and pass the nice nurse the scan disk and biopsy report.

"I'll have the doctor take a look at these and then he'll be right in." She smiled and immediately left.

"They seem so professional." I'm totally smiling and completely happy that I'm in THIS hospital and THESE are the people that are going to help me. The second the surgeon in Laconia said 'Uh…yeah…you need to go to Boston,' I was completely relieved and now that I am here I feel like I can actually breathe! I feel like I'm not going to be sucked beneath the surface of the deep, dank water in the bottom of the Canterbury well. I'm not running through the dark and dangerous forest as fast and furiously as I can, while heavy footsteps are charging after me. I'm not about to be carried out to sea atop a giant tidal wave that nobody saw coming. I'm holding my head up and above the surface and I'm breathing! And the water is massaging my entire body as I continue to float and swim through the warm salty embrace of the ocean.

"They ARE the professionals." Albert's the one smirking now like he knew it the whole time but had elected to say nothing until this very moment when of course it is now completely obvious.

"You have crumbs on your lips." I'm laughing inside of my head at the thought of the nice nurse who must have noticed that Albert had obviously been stuffing his face with free muffins and pastry in the first waiting room. "How can you not feel that?" I'm shaking my head at him now as he quickly rubs his lips together in an effort to remove the evidence before the doctor comes into the examination room.

"Hello, how are you?" A very pleasant man with a long white medical coat suddenly swings open the door and I immediately recognize him as one of the Thoracic surgeons from the hospital website. The surgeon in Laconia had initially asked me if I knew any of the doctors here and I remember sitting in silence as my mind got stuck with that question. How the hell would I just happen to know a surgeon from a top medical center/hospital in Boston? Eventually I merely said that I was confident there would be no bad choices; the surgeon chuckled and had his nurse schedule me to meet with the very surgeon I am now meeting.

"Hello." I'm smiling. I'm thrilled to meet this man. I'm thrilled to hear that nothing is really wrong with me!

Oh my GOD, did I just think that? DAMMIT! I thought my mind had gotten through that part!!! Am I truly still stuck way back at the beginning of this entire misguided adventure? The adventure that has done nothing but piss me off from the second Brad called and told me to find a primary care physician and get the 'something's there' followed up on? The adventure that has done nothing up until this point but scare the ever living shit out of me and provided me with no answers whatsoever about what the hell I am supposed to do if any or all of these useless and expensive medical tests are actually semi or partially correct! What the hell is going on with me and why can I not get my head around any of this freaking information?!

It's because the information is not right! The information is incorrect! The freaking tests, scans, x-rays and biopsies were all done by a huge group of incompetent cheerleaders who know absolutely nothing about what they are doing, which is why they freaking sent me here in the freaking first place! And I swear to Christ when I get the astronomical medical bill that for some reason my insurance company will deny because the tests and appointments were all completely unnecessary, I will go ape shit on somebody's ass!

"Why are you here?" He's still smiling.

I knew it! I knew nothing was wrong! Just like when we

took our second born into the hospital because the doctor was worried that his skull plates had fused too soon and the first thing the doctor at that hospital said to me was 'why are you here?' And he said that because he was confused. He was confused because after he (the true professional) looked at the results of the useless and waste of money medical tests, he couldn't figure out why on earth we were wasting his time because there was absolutely nothing wrong with our child! I knew it!!

The incredibly smart surgeon person that is sitting across the room from me right now is going to clear everything up and he's going to tell me that the lab-rat in the Laconia hospital must have compromised the cells they ripped out of my body during the biopsy. That person (lab-rat) must have been eating lunch while performing the tests on my cells. He must have dropped a crumb that had clung to his lips, like the crumbs that Albert just licked from his lips, into the test-tube of my cells thereby causing a false positive result for cancer! He's going to tell me that the tumors are actually quite normal and often people live their entire lives without even realizing that they have them. He's going to tell me that the tumors pose no threat whatsoever but I should probably keep an eye on them and he'll send a report to my primary care physician! I knew nothing was wrong this whole time! I KNEW IT!!!

"Are you here for a second opinion or treatment?" Before I could even spit out a single word the surgeon continued with the second half of his question and I could feel my soul begin to sink again. My mind stopped. My mind just stared straight ahead at the incredibly smart surgeon person sitting in front of me. I was shifting backwards and I felt my entire being suddenly re-reverting to the state of zombification.

"Treatment." I responded after a momentary pause as the surgeon just politely waited for my zombie mind to compute that I'd actually just been asked a question. I'm continuing to just stare straight ahead and I'm completely positive I can feel drool dripping down my chin from my flopping zombie bottom lip.

"Okay." The smile vanished from the surgeon's face. He spun around on his chair and looked at the computer back to me and back to the computer again. He was studying slide after slide of my torso and the swirls of black, gray and white tissue photos.

I smiled at him and braced myself.

"I've taken a look at your scan." He's so pleasant even though he's being serious. I can tell by the way he's speaking that he knows exactly what he's talking about. He hasn't even said anything yet but he's impressing me that his mind is extremely intelligent. He's one of those people that you meet and you can just tell that they are a complete genius.

"Okay." I intently listen as the surgeon that's a complete genius took me through a complete explanation of my body. He told me that there's a lining around my lungs that folds back over and onto itself again. Sort of like a balloon. If you blew up a balloon and then pressed your fist into it; part of the balloon would directly connect to the surface of your hand and the other part would be over and around your hand sort of like a sandwich of balloon and air. Well the balloon is the pleura lining around my lung and the hand is in fact my lung. I chuckled at the description but could now understand how my body is actually put together. And then the surgeon spun back around and pulled the computer screen around so we could all see it together. He showed me the same scans that we'd already looked at before with the surgeon in Laconia. And he showed me multiple tumors that have for some reason grown and have now appeared within the pleura lining around my right lung. I was nodding and smiling as the surgeon taught me and Albert and showed us where and what the 'something's there' are. The more the surgeon talked and explained what was going on, the more I felt my state of zombification ease. The surgeon is a teacher. And the lesson he is taking Albert and I through right now is more information and explanation than we have received this entire time full of weeks of tests, Brad from the Orthopedic Center, more tests and a new primary care physician, more tests, a surgeon and more tests and the surgeon again but this time with his entourage of nurses which included the military nurse and the giant man nurse. And when the lesson was complete the incredibly smart surgeon rolled his chair away from the computer completely and looked at me directly.

And then he said it. And he said it with confidence. In one little tiny sentence the surgeon gave me exactly what I needed.

"The tumors need to come out."

Chapter 24

OKAY!! I have a plan!

NOW I can get my head around the fact that I actually have an issue. Now that the professional and incredibly smart surgeon from one of the BIG hospitals has told me what I need to do, I can hold my head above the splashing waters that threatened to drown me only moments ago!

"Here we go!" I'm bouncing up and down in my seat as Albert once again attempts to get us back through the traffic of Boston and onto the road which leads to where we live. Even though I feel like I have not been living anywhere for more than a few months now; now that I have a plan I feel like I can live! Now I know what I am supposed to do and I can actually write it on the calendar! (Yes...I'm still one of those people that writes appointments onto a paper calendar, versus typing them into a virtual calendar program thing in the bowels of my freaking cell phone that pisses me off every time it ring-sings)

"Just don't talk." Albert's propped up on the front edge of his seat with his face smashed into the windshield again.

"I need to call my mother." I'm excited.

"Not until we get to the highway." He's chomping on a piece of gum like it's stuck so far into his teeth that the gum is threatening to overtake his sinus cavities and jawbone, and the more ferociously he chomps the more stuck the gum becomes between the cracks of his freaking bone sized freaking teeth! Jesus Christ can he please just get onto the same page with me?? Why can't his mind just connect with my very thoughts at exactly the moment that I need him to do just that?!!!

And then I remember when he saved me from drowning in the bottom of the Canterbury well, and I decide to sit silently until he manages to get us to the highway.

I'm glad Albert is with me for this trip to the chaotic big city that makes us both feel like pikes out of water. I'm glad that he's there to listen to everything that the doctor tells me to do. Because I am certainly going to be sitting on the ugly couch at the off season rental cottage this evening when I turn toward Albert and ask him 'what exactly did the doctor say?' My brain was celebrating the minute the doctor gave me a plan. The minute I heard the confidence in his voice and the instruction and the direction regarding surgery I was good. I nodded my head and I smiled the entire time he was telling me about the plan. I agreed to everything the doctor said without so much as a question, request for clarification, or inquisitive frown. And I truly had no reason to question anything really; because in my mind the expert is going to decide what I am going to do. The expert is the one that in my mind gets to decide what I am going to go through because the expert is the only one that understands what is going on. He's the one that has been there and done that. He's the one that has experienced and managed a project like the one that has been bestowed to me. So why would I question him? He's one of the best in the world. What he says goes! I'm good! I only need to hear him say what it is that he's going to do and then I'm completely and one hundred percent on board and ready to go!

Albert asked a question. Albert asked him about our upcoming family vacation trip to Puerto Rico that we scheduled nearly one year ago. He asked him because of scheduling because obviously he knows I intend to go on the vacation. Albert and the doctor looked at the calendar and they scheduled me for surgery. I nodded my head and said that it was fine. It has to be. The tumors need to come out. I have a plan.

And when we are at 'home' this evening and I ask Albert what the doctor said, THEN I will begin to comprehend what my body will be going through. When Albert explains that the surgeon is going to make four incisions across the side and back of my rib cage, deflate my right lung, peel off the outer layer of the clear plasma membrane thing that surrounds my freaking lung, cut, burn, seal and build it all back together, re-inflate my lung and stitch the skin back in place after having removed the alien being fucking tumor that has decided to set up camp around an organ that I happen to need to survive…I'll realize what exactly is about to happen!

But for now.

I need to move into my new home.

Unpack.

Work at my new job.

Explain to my children that everything is going to be okay.
Breathe.
Call my mother.
Go on VACATION!
Keep my head above the water while I continue to swim!
And just try to FUCKING relax!

Chapter 25

Today is the day that our first load of furniture arrives! Albert left the off-season rental cottage before the crack of dawn with our second oldest son and by the time I get out of work they should have arrived back in town with a giant truck load of our stuff. Tomorrow we have a couple of friends and three of our children helping to unload. Fortunately I have the weekend off so I will spend my time unpacking and putting together some of our new home! Hopefully it's only going to be two giant truck loads; the goal is to have everything in the house by the end of the weekend. I can't wait to settle in! I can't wait to feel like my feet are back on the ground! I can't wait to sleep in my own bed and cook a meal in my own kitchen! And all of this will happen just in time for my family to come together for the reunion in Puerto Rico! And the second day after I return from our wonderful vacation I head to the giant hospital in Boston for 'The Plan'!!!

It doesn't even matter to me that everything in my life seems to happen at exactly the same moment. Everything seems to shatter against the wall as if I've just thrown a crystal glass vase across the room. And the glass has exploded into a thousand splinters and filled the room with shards of flesh cutting tiny spears, forcing me to dart, twist and turn as I tiptoe around the broken glass. None of that matters to me at all because when everything happens at the same time that is when I feel myself charging full speed ahead! That is when I am being forced to proceed because it is the only way for me to keep up with that which is happening all around me. That is when my soul can truly run! This is when my mind can focus on the tasks at hand and just get things done because if I stop for even a moment to think about everything that is happening I might get scared. If I get scared my 'running full speed ahead' will suddenly become 'running away'. So I'd rather just be crazy busy so I can keep from turning into just plain crazy! I need to just do this!

"Good morning!" I'm practically singing as I walk past the tongue flickering snake. She's never happy to see me. She never seems to smile about anything. And her eyes are nothing but slits as she tightens her lips and stares at me as I walk past her after entering the store.

"Hi." She hisses her idea of a greeting at me which is no kind of greeting at all. Her saying 'Hi' sounds like she's spitting venom directly into my eyes as her tongue continues to flicker.

"Isn't it beautiful outside today?" I'm smiling. She says absolutely nothing as she turns and slithers through the women's department away from me. Her body is crooked and her torso is tipped slightly forward as she moves with a slow gliding motion.

On the short trip to the back of the building and into my office I once again witness injured associates. They are laying along the side of the departments with visible wounds still fresh with blood, where the snake has plunged her filthy fangs deeply into their flesh. And as I passed by them they quickly told me the stories. They told me exactly how she had treated them on that very morning. And the more I heard the more I knew exactly what the future holds for the tongue flickering snake that lurks throughout the women's department. She will be gone!

Quietly I closed the door to my office and called my boss.

"Good morning!" Wow, he sounds happy to hear from me for some reason.

"Hi. I'm sorry to bother you but I wanted to give you an update since my appointment with the Boston surgeon." I'm pleasant but I'm nervous. My boss doesn't know me and I'm sure he's expecting more than what he's about to receive from me.

"Oh that's right! What did he say?" Really? Did he actually forget that I have been diagnosed with cancer? He must have thought I was just calling to give him fabulous news about the store and results. And why on earth did he just assume that my surgeon is a man? He is but that's not even the point!

"I'm going to be having surgery." I'm pausing. I'm waiting for some sort of statement. Something like 'I'm so sorry you have to go through that but don't worry everything will be okay.' And the pause went on and on to the point that I thought we'd disconnected. "Are you still there?"

"How long are you going to be out for?" Wow. He's actually angry. I can hear it in his voice and I'm suddenly wishing I'd just sent him an email.

"I don't know. At least a couple of months, I would

imagine."

"Well, what's the surgery for?" Seriously?? He has NO right to even ask me that question! Medical details are not something that I am obligated to provide and he should know that he cannot make requests for private information! Who the hell is this guy anyway?

"They are going to remove the pleura lining from around my right lung." I don't mind giving the information and am actually the type of person that is pretty open and forthcoming with details. I would have told him anyway. Again, it's not the point!

"What?!"

"That's where the tumors are." More silence from him. More pausing. I'll bet he's rubbing his forehead and wishing he'd never hired me. He doesn't know me so he doesn't really care about me as a person. He's focusing on the store and HIS numbers, which amount to HIS bonus at the end of the year. And I can't even really hold it against him because his demands for results are truly a prerequisite for his position. It's who he is and what he does.

"When?" I can hear him breathing hard and I know it's NOT because he's crying. He's steaming!

"The second day after I arrive home from Puerto Rico."

"You're still taking that vacation?!" Now he is practically yelling.

"Yes." Again with the silence. Again with a long pause. He's formulating his next question and struggling to control himself. I wonder what he really wants to say to me. Probably something like 'you're not going to be here for a couple of months and you feel you should still take your vacation?' He quickly must realize that once again he's made an error; he cannot demand that I not take my earned time off.

"Wow. I'm just surprised your doctor will allow you to fly and go so far away." Nice save.

"There's no issue with flying; my husband made sure to ask the surgeon. And the trip is a family reunion trip; there are thirty family members going. All five of my children are going and we've planned this for a year. It's important, especially now, that I spend this time with my children and my husband. And it's not even a reason but oh by the way I've already shelled out more than five-thousand dollars for the plane tickets, rented condo and car."

"I understand." Now he's starting to sound more human. Perhaps my statement of 'especially now' is what it took to sink into his numbers driven head that I am facing a major surgery and my family is probably scared to death that I'm going to freaking die! Or perhaps he's talking about the non-refundable five-thousand dollars I'd lose if I cancelled. "You need to call Benefits and fill out all the forms."

"I'll do it today." Now I'm starting to relax. The news is delivered. My boss knows the plan. And it is what it is. There's no discussion that needs to happen.

"Okay. How's everything else?" He sounds tired now. His day is just beginning and I've already exhausted him.

"I'm going to have to put my second assistant on a performance plan. She continues to abuse the staff. It needs to stop. I have multiple statements from multiple associates that I'll be forwarding to you and corporate."

"You can't do anything with you going out on medical. We need her just to run the store right now. You'll have to just deal with her when you get back."

"Oh?" I can't believe that is the direction he's just given me in regard to the snake. Leave her alone and let her continue to strike and spit into the eyes of every single associate in the building? Let her continue to sink her fangs into their flesh? Let her continue to lurk in the shadows of the building, terrorizing all that wander through the departments? Is he kidding?!

"Yes. OH!" He's angry again. Perhaps being NOT allowed to address the snake's behavior is my punishment for having to go out on medical leave. "I'm pulling into another store so need to go. Keep me posted." And then he just hung up.

It's official! I have become the 'pain in the ass' manager within the entire district. I'm the one that pisses off my boss every time I call. I'm the one that was supposed to be amazing but instead has become a huge disappointment and I've somehow managed to do it in record time! And unfortunately my boss is also a pain in the ass and not at all the supportive and genuine person that I thought he was going to be when I first met him! This is a recipe for failure and completely NOT what I had in mind when I relocated my entire family to New Hampshire. BUT then again I also was not planning to get cancer!

As I hung up the telephone I immediately began to think about the snake. My wheels are turning and I'm preparing for what I WILL do whether my boss likes it or not! I refuse to allow the snake to continue to strike! I might not be able to officially address her behavior but I can certainly let her know how inappropriate it is. I can continue with the trail of documented conversations which I will need anyway when I officially begin to push her incompetent evil ass out of the building the second I return from my medical leave!

As the snake continues to flicker her tongue and lurk throughout the shadows of the women's department, I begin to envision the snare which she will most assuredly find herself snagged in, even after my departure for a medical leave.

Chapter 26

The day is finally here! We are actually moving into our new home! Albert did a phenomenal job with the painting, flooring and cleaning! Just a few moments after I left work for the day and bid the snake goodbye, Albert called me and said he's just one exit south of where we live. He should be pulling into the driveway in about fifteen more minutes. And as I stand in the clean, freshly painted house waiting for him and my son to pull into the driveway I begin to stroll. I'm walking in a giant circle through the first floor of our three level home. And it's so quiet in here. There's not another single person in the house with me and this might very well be the only time I am completely and utterly alone in my new home. The dog isn't even here yet. She's hiding underneath the bed in the very back bedroom of the off-season rental cottage. And the house that I'm standing in is already clean and ready for our stuff to be marched in, armload after armload after armload.

The paint in the kitchen is a beautiful shade of sage green and the cupboards are cream colored. The living room is a soft caramel color with off-white trim around the windows. The floors are a combination of large white tiles and medium brown hardwood of some sort. And the entire first floor is one big giant open room that houses the kitchen, eating area, office and living room. I would be able to pedal around on a bicycle in here right now if I actually owned one because there is just so much space!

The kitchen sits at the very back of the larger than large room which is the entire first floor. And right next to where the dining table and chairs will sit is a giant window that overlooks the waterfront. And as I stare out the huge window I can already imagine our birdhouse and wind chimes dangling from the low branches in the one tree that grows in the narrow backyard. Across the water just a tiny ways is a horseshoe shaped island. There are signs that appear to be posted here and there along the edge of the island that demand boaters to NOT create any wakes as they float by what is truly a sanctuary for thousands of birds. Just staring out the window I wonder if every passing motorist that I hear is actually Albert with the moving truck. I can't wait for him to get here and I can't wait to march box after box into our home. I already feel like I am starting to breathe again.

And I find myself thinking about my bed. My great big king size glorious bed that I haven't been able to sleep in for so many months now. I imagine my bed which will sit in the room that is directly above the kitchen next to an identical window to the one that I'm looking out right now except that it is on the second floor of the house. That window and all of its enormity will be the window that I will gaze out and over the horseshoe shaped island as I'm recovering from surgery in just a couple of weeks. That is the window that I will watch the flurry of cardinals, king fishers, eagles, sparrows, robins, great blue herons and chickadees to just name a mere few of the thousands of birds that live here. That is the window that I will watch the clouds roll over the mountains that sit way off in the distance along the horizon behind an old white steeple church on the other side of the water. And perhaps I'll watch some severe thunderstorms stretch and clap across the low lying dark clouds at the end of a scorching hot ninety degree summer day.

In the Fall I'll look out the massive window in my bedroom and I'll see the amazing colors of the leaves as they begin to turn. The Maple and Quaking Aspen will change first, quickly followed by the Oaks and Ash. And the colors will be so incredible. If there are any people in this world that have never seen the beauty of a New England Fall and the glory of the changing colors of the trees, they really just need to take a trip and come to see what I will get to watch from my glorious king size bed. And as I imagine what those colors of coral, neon yellow, deep red, and brilliant orange will be like I breathe so deeply and I close my eyes before exhaling quietly.

And when I open my eyes again I find myself thinking about the winters. What about the snow? The snow will be just as beautiful as the glorious colors of the leaves. There will be many opportunities to watch the flakes fly ferociously and then again sometimes they will just float all around the atmosphere like we are all living within a giant snow globe. The flakes will land along every single crook and cranny of every single leafless branch of the single tree in the narrow backyard along the edge of the water.

My entire world will be so incredibly clean and crisp and glowing white on every morning following the snow. And as much as we all get annoyed because we have to deal with the snow and drive through it and shovel it and have things cancel because of it; I can't imagine living without it. I can't imagine living without getting such opportunities to witness such immense beauty with all of its whiteness. And with my thoughts I suddenly find myself hugging my very own person, hanging my head, and once again closing my eyes. I don't even remember breathing as I stood and thought of my bed and my body curled up in it as I watched the ever changing seasons of my life. Then I slowly opened my eyes as I heard the roaring grumble of the moving truck backing into the driveway that runs along the very side of the kitchen, dining, office and living room. And I only had a moment before the door would fly open and my husband and second born will be standing there wearing a layer of dust, with looks of complete exhaustion. And the moment was all it took for my brain to make an almighty leap into the harshest of all the realities I've ever had to face within my mere fifty years of life.

What will happen if I don't?

What will happen if I never get to lay in my bed and look out the giant window with vast appreciation for the changing of the seasons?

What will happen if I don't lay and watch the flurry of the thousands of birds that live on the horse shoe shaped island?

What will happen if I don't smile with stunning appreciation for the amazing colors of the changing leaves?

And what will happen if I don't get up in the morning and need to block the glare from my eyes as I stare in wonderment at the brilliance of newly fallen snow?

What is going to happen if none of what I imagine and yearn for does not in fact ever happen?

Slowly I slumped forward and slowly I began to move backward and slowly I tiptoed away from the giant window that sits at the very back of the first floor of our new home. Quietly I clasped my hands together and held them against the front of my breasts with the very tip of my fingers gently touching my bottom lip. My eyes are closed and my breathing is shallow. I can feel my bottom lip starting to quiver and there's an immense pressure at the bottom of my throat as I struggle to hold my thoughts together. I'm struggling to move my thoughts past the incredible fear that is overtaking the gentleness of the scenes playing out through the giant window in the kitchen of my new home. I can hear the footsteps of my husband and son as they trudge toward the side doorway from the driveway. They will be standing directly behind me in just a moment. And I don't want them to see my struggle. I don't want them to feel badly when they see the tears welling up in my eyes. I don't want to burden them with my fears and my thoughts of 'what if.' I need to swallow hard and I need to just pretend that everything is going to be okay because for all I really know it will be. I need help! I just need to get through this for the sake of my family! I need to keep my thoughts together and I need to stop losing my grip on the fact that everything is going to be okay! I'm going to be okay but I am so completely terrified that for one reason or another something is going to go wrong and I will in fact not be okay! Anything could happen! Anything can happen when I'm laid out on that operating table and the surgeon deflates my lung. What if I stop breathing? What if my blood pressure suddenly falls so sharply that they are unable to get it back up? What if my heart stops beating?!!! What if I bleed to death?!!! What if I have a severe reaction to some drug that they give me that is supposed to actually help me to get through the procedure but it in fact does the exact opposite and freaking kills me?!!!

I need to stop this thinking! I have the best doctors in the world. They've done this before! Christ, they're probably the ones that invented the surgery that I'm about to have! They know what they're doing and they are going to make sure that I will be okay! I need to relax. I need to just keep my head on straight and focus on the good news. They found the 'something's there' and they're going to get it out of me and I'm going to be just fine!

And then I finally breathe.

I breathe just as the side door in the kitchen swings open and my husband and second born are standing there looking at me. I smiled at them as I silently prayed.

'Oh, my God…

…

… Please don't let me die.'

Chapter 27

This morning is another new day!

Fortunately Albert and Thomas unloaded the entire truck by themselves. Apparently truck number one was completely full of everything that lives in the basement of our new home. And that everything includes every single tool for auto mechanics and every single tool needed for home construction. The one thing that we really need with any house that we ever live in but unfortunately didn't get with this particular house is a garage. Albert needs an entire building for all of his things that live inside of the basement. And most of the things that live inside of the basement required both Albert and Thomas to lift together because of the bulk and weight of the things. I got out of the entire unload of truck number one. Once the unloading began last evening, I basically was put in charge of sandwiches, chips and soda; which I am completely fine with and actually somewhat relieved!

And this morning before I even woke up in the off season rental cottage, Albert and Thomas were already gone again with the empty truck. Back down to Massachusetts where they will load up with the final two storage units before heading back this way. By the time they get here my two youngest daughters will have arrived straight from the college dorm. Albert's brother and best friend who lives in Maine also went to Massachusetts to help Albert load the truck. Eventually we will all head to the new house and together we will unload of all of the stuff that will most assuredly fill every room of our new home.

I haven't seen my girls since we all found out that I have cancer. In fact the only one of my five children that has been home since the news hit, has been Thomas. And Thomas is so genuine and caring that when he looked at me and asked for the answer to it all, I found myself believing exactly what I told him.

"You're going to be okay, right?" He said.

"Yes! I'll be fine. This is just a pain in my ass and something that we have to deal with."

It was what he needed to hear and it was what I TRULY do believe! In my heart I just feel like everything is going to be okay.

I know that I am going to die someday just like the rest of us, but I also KNOW that today is not that day! And neither is tomorrow and neither is the day of my surgery! So why do I find myself still getting knocked over by a tidal wave of emotions, fears and fits of 'begging for forgiveness' from the Almighty? Why do I find that my thoughts are as scattered as the flocking birds that live on the horse shoe shaped island? Why can't I have ONE thought and just stay with that thought for even one single freaking day?!

It's an awful thing when your own swirling thoughts and emotions are completely exhausting to your own mind! Because you can't just punch out and go home to get away from your thoughts. You can't tell your thoughts that you have plans and need to reschedule the lunch you thought you'd be able to tolerate with them. You can't see your thoughts from across the room and suddenly dart behind the tall plant and hope that your thoughts didn't see you. Your thoughts are like the controllers. You can try to reason with them. You can try to make promises to them. You can swear to them that you will never eat another drop of anything that contains preservatives, you will never smoke another cigarette or really classy slim-lined girly cigar, you will never heat any food in the microwave especially if it's in plastic, or you will never absolutely NEVER live in a house that has basement full of cracks that leak clouds of invisible putrid radon odorless even though we all know it's there GAS!!! But no matter how much you plead with your thoughts to just give you some legitimacy they will not. No matter how much you bargain with them in the hopes that your thoughts will just let you relax for a moment so you perhaps can sleep, eat and breathe like a 'normal' person, they will not. Your thoughts can be fooled perhaps for a moment or two on a day that you are really busy with things that take your thoughts away from the scary realities. Your thoughts can be teased and taunted enough that they look away from you for a second, like the dog you pretend to throw a ball for. But your thoughts are smarter than you think. They never forget. They will return. They will be back. And the more they return and begin to take control again, the more you begin to realize that all of your bargaining, teasing and pleading is truly in vain. Our thoughts have learned how to manipulate us. They have learned to persuade us because they always know what we're thinking. They're a very tricky bunch and could probably rule the world if they set your mind to it.

But the fact of the matter is that our thoughts are actually NOT the one in control. Thoughts are how we process. Thoughts are how we get through it. Thoughts are how we learn to accept the situation and formulate a plan for dealing with it. The real trick is to realize just exactly that and the sooner we all realize that, the sooner we can just focus on the task at hand! Because life and what happens within our world is truly a task. The things that happen to us are 'things' that we just have to figure out how to manage. This is a project. It's a project that I need to manage.

Just like my thoughts blurted out the response to Thomas and I meant it. 'This is just a pain in my ass and something we are going to have to deal with.' For whatever reason I have cancer. Maybe it's because I smoked? Maybe it's because I ate too many packaged cupcakes and processed food? Maybe I played in a sandbox that was full of radioactive dirt that some giant company had infested and then 'filled' into a giant hole at the end of the street that I grew up on? Maybe it's in my genes? The answer to the burning question that I'll never find an answer for doesn't really even matter after all. I have it. Now I have to just deal with it.

And what in the hell does 'deal with it' even mean? Why did I have to say that to Thomas? Isn't that obvious? Isn't that what everybody does? Doesn't anybody that is diagnosed with cancer go to the doctor and follow the instructions? Or are there people out there that just don't? Are there people out there that give up? Are there people out there that are content with the news? Are there people out there that find out they have lung cancer and then decide to just keep smoking three packs a day because the fact that they now have cancer was just their destiny anyways and they actually enjoy smoking more than living?

I enjoyed smoking! I loved it! In fact....truth be told I was secretly still smoking right up until Brad called and said that they found the 'something's there'. I was secretly opening the tiny window in the living room of the off-season rental cottage and smoking a cigarette that I continually blew fast and furiously through the screen, all the while being terrified that one of the owner's meddling neighbors would catch me and turn me in because the cottage I rented was non-smoking! And I didn't care!

And I loved it! I smoked two entire cigarettes every single evening in the off-season rental cottage! Every night it was so freaking cold when I opened the tiny window and I shivered as I secretly smoked and smoked before Albert and Thomas and the dog arrived! And I'd do it again because for all I know the cancer came from the packaged freaking cupcakes!!!

But none of that matters anyway because I have cancer now. What has happened already cannot be changed but how I manage the project in front of me can change the outcome of the hand I've been dealt for whatever the reason truly happens to be. It is what it is. Now what I do from here is all that matters. More importantly…I am NOT going to die! Just yet, anyways.

Is it okay to say 'die' if you truly do not believe that it will be because of what is happening right now? Is 'die' like a four letter word even though it only has three? If I use it in a sentence when I'm speaking with my children are they going to freak right the hell out because I said the D-word?

My thoughts have become the flocking of the birds again…

Where the hell are my two youngest?

It's already two o'clock in the afternoon. I'm sitting here in this freaking off-season rental cottage waiting for them, waiting for the call that truck number two is just around the corner, as I just continue to battle with my thoughts while I stare at the dog. And I'm already drinking wine!

I'm not giving up the wine!

There's no proof that wine causes cancer!

Christ, I hope there's not!

Chapter 28

The girls arrived as scheduled and we had just enough time to pick up pizza, chips, packaged cupcakes and drinks on our way over to the new house from the off season rental cottage. As soon as we pulled into the driveway Albert was coming around the corner with the truck full of stuff. And behind him was his brother and his best friend from Maine. Thank God for their support because without them I am completely positive that the oak armoire in my bedroom would have never made it up the stairs!

Throughout the afternoon we resembled a sort of manufacturing plant. Items continually flowing around and around and up the stairs, back down and out of the house again to gather another armful of stuff, back into the house and over and over again. We were a well-oiled machine by the end of the final unloading event. And when the truck was completely empty we immediately began to fill it up again with stuff that we suddenly realized we never should have packed, put into storage, put into the moving truck and unloaded into the new house. The final step of the entire moving process amounted to numerous trips to the local Salvation Army store where Albert and I have been dubbed 'Donators of the Month'. And 'yes' we should have done this before we packed, stored and hauled the things that we are donating but Albert was the only person that had been burdened with the arduous task of packing. I was already here and living in the hotel room and then the off season rental cottage. Albert didn't want to accidentally get rid of things that I might truly still want to keep. He did the right thing. But WOW, what a pile of donations!

Finally our friend from Maine and Albert's brother were driving away and we were suddenly alone as a partial family in our new home. Finally I was going to be able to sleep in my own bed. Finally I was going to be able to relax. And as we all sat in the living room, eating left-over pizza I found myself just thinking and staring at my two youngest daughters as they chewed their dinner and tapped incessantly on their cell-phones.

I don't think they get it. I don't think my daughters understand what is happening to me. They seem oblivious. They almost roll their eyes every time I bring up the whole cancer thing. And I swear to God the only comment I can even recall them making when we originally spoke about everything was, 'Oh, Mom. You'll be fine.' And today on the drive over from the off season rental cottage they asked me if we would have time to go shopping while they're here. And it's not like I'm looking to see them cry or stress about my upcoming surgery and the fact that the C-word has invaded our lives but I'm worried that if something does go wrong their heads will completely implode when they hear the news. They are not connecting with this. It's either that or they really don't even give a shit and it absolutely just cannot be that! They are my daughters for goodness sake and I know they love me. I can't figure out what is going on with them and I don't want to harass them about it just because I don't understand how they are processing things.

Or perhaps it's just me? Am I acting all ridiculous because I'm nervous about having surgery? Is it really NOT a big deal at all and I'm acting stupid or something? Is the whole thing going to be as simple as a magician pulling a hidden scarf out of his sleeve, when the surgeon magically removes the pleura lining from my right lung? Is the pleura-thing just floating around in there as if it were in outer space and all the doctor needs to do is grab just a tiny little piece of its corner, yank really hard and voila! Suddenly the surgery is over and the cancer is all gone now? Maybe it's just like pulling a table cloth out from underneath an entire setting of dishes? And when I wake up in my room after the surgery I'll feel as if I've only taken a quick nap and perhaps just pulled a muscle or two on my side. It's just going to hurt for a few days but then I'll be back to work in no time, right?

What am I worried about? What the hell is wrong with me? Why am I the only one that's cried? Why am I the only one that is spending any time at all dwelling and thinking about this horribly scary and dangerous procedure that I am actually going to have to force myself to go through, even though I don't want to, but I really don't have any choice because we/I am dealing with having freaking cancer! And this was not the plan! This was not what I had in mind when I moved my entire family to the great State of New Hampshire so I could start the job that I've been working to get promoted into for more than five years now! Why did this have to happen? Why am I being forced to go through this? What did I do wrong? Why does this have to happen to me? And why the hell can't anybody hear me screaming about this within the walls of my fragile and terrified mind?!

Just when I feel like I've wrapped my thoughts around everything that's positive and resembling fields full of flying fuzz, butterflies and pixies, my mind suddenly snaps back into the dark and dangerous corners full of spiders and bats in the deepest recesses of a horrific and unexplored cave. And I'm walking as slow as I possibly can through the cave. And the ceiling is so high that I can't even tip my head far enough back to see the very top of the incredibly huge yet hidden hole. I can't for the life of me realize how I got here and I can't for the life of me figure out how to find my way out of this horrific cave. I'm stuck and I'm completely and utterly lost. I'm spinning in circles and I'm flailing my arms as I try to feel my way along a cold and dripping rock wall. There are corners and crevices and the constant tap-tap-tapping of dripping water that is falling from the incredibly tall ceiling to pools of murky stank-filled water that's run through the abandoned paths of rock within the floor of the cave. As hard as I'm struggling to focus and see through the darker than dark thick stank air, I cannot. I'm moving and flailing randomly and hoping that I will suddenly be able to see just a smidgeon of light coming through the tiniest of the cracks along the darkest of all of the walls within the cave. And that light will be the way for me to find my way out of the deep dark stench filled cave that somehow I've wandered into and become completely and utterly lost!

"Mom?"

One of the twins is staring at me as I lift my eyes from my stale slice of pizza and gaze into her beautiful dark brown eyes.

"Mom?"

"What?" Did she see me struggling? Did she notice when I was simply staring at nothing while my mind was struggling to find my way through the darker than dark cave? Does she know that I need her? Does she know that I feel completely and utterly alone right now and I desperately need somebody to tell me that it's going to be okay for real? Does she know that I'm about to burst? My feelings and my fears are at the highest and most vulnerable level of desperation that I've ever experienced in my entire life and I feel as if I've lost complete control as I flail and spin within the treacherous walls of the horrific cave! Is she going to save me? Is she going to smile and tell me that I'm going to be just fine because for some reason she truly does in fact know that it will really be okay? "What is it, Honey?"

Innocently she looked back at me. Her face is still round and adorable and the dimple on her right cheek looks exactly the same as the one on Albert's cheek. She looks exactly the same to me as the day she probably first formulated a true sentence and asked a similar question of her mother and she was probably a mere two years old. She's my daughter and she's innocent and even though she's now an adult, she's still oblivious. Even after all these years she still does not realize that sometimes the monsters underneath the bed can still scare us.

"Do we have any juice?"

I smiled as I stood up and walked toward the refrigerator. My daughters are exactly like Albert. They all think I'm Superman.

Chapter 29

My last day of work before my vacation begins! Almost my last day of work before heading off to the hospital to have my lung peeled apart; but I can't even focus on that right now. I'm only going to focus on the vacation part of my life right now! I packed my bag as soon as I unpacked my clothes last evening and I cannot believe that in less than twenty-four hours I'll be on a plane headed for Puerto Rico! I just have to get through today and am already planning on leaving work early. My entire day will be spent in my office as I organize, email and instruct my team on how to handle things and who's in charge of what in my absence.

"You wanted to see me?" The snake is standing in the doorway.

"Yes. Close the door and have a seat please." I motion for her to enter.

"Okay." Her voice is quiet. Her tone is innocent. And I realize what a good actress she is because there is nothing quiet and innocent about her behavior and personality. She's trying to come across as a sweet person just by raising the inflection in her voice. It's not going to work. I can hear the flicker of her tongue as she quietly closes the door before turning back around to face me. "How are you doing?" She asks as she slinks into one of the guest chairs in my office.

"I'm fine." If she thinks I'm going to have a conversation with her like we're friends she is sadly mistaken. I've already told her about my medical plans and there's no update to share. My conversations with the snake consist of nothing more than facts. I'm not interested in sharing my feelings or my life with an evil intending serpent. "The reason I wanted to talk to you is because I'm getting some feedback about you from some of the associates."

"Oh?" She's acting surprised; as if she's never dreamed that an associate could possibly have anything negative to say about her.

Briefly and professionally I explained to the snake that she needs to change her behavior and the entire time I was speaking I watched her contort her face, as she closed her eyes more and more until they became two incredulous slits of light within the dark creviced face of a serpent. She said nothing further beyond the initial 'Oh?' and most importantly she denied nothing. She knew that the news was true; she knew because that is her nature of actions and they were being called out with too many examples and direct quotes from her fellow associates who had reached their breaking point. They turned her in and she was busted. I explained to her in detail many examples and there were many different people that had stepped forward to say that they no longer wanted to live with the fear of being struck down by the lurking serpent that hid amongst the fixtures of clothing within the store. And when the conversation, which was more like a speech, was over she had heard a full explanation of what I would not tolerate from her ever but especially in my absence. Her skin was red and blotched across her neck and cheeks and her slits for eyes were bloodshot. In silence she stood back up and slithered from my office. She offered me no explanation beyond a quick nod of her head and a flicker of her tongue. The message was delivered and that was all I would be allowed to do for the entire team of good hearted individuals that work for me before my medical leave begins. It would have to be enough for now.

The remainder of my final day of work before vacation was spent cleaning up lingering emails, schedule requests and leaving my management team, including the snake, instructions for who needs to be doing what while I am gone. When I walked out of the building at the end of my day the air was so warm and the wind was so gentle, I immediately felt relaxed and ready for a week with my family in a tropical paradise!

Chapter 30

Oh my God, today is the day! I was so excited when the alarm clock sounded off at a mere four o'clock in the morning that I practically leapt out of bed. I felt like a child on Christmas morning running through the halls, up the stairs to the third floor, knocking on bedroom doors and telling everybody to wake up because it was time! It was the kind of morning that took forever to arrive and from the second my head hit my pillow last evening I just laid in my bed anticipating the screaming buzz of the alarm telling me to hurry up and get to the airport! It was finally time! Time to fly from our beds, throw the already packed suitcases into the back of the giant big man car and get on the highway! In just one half of a day we would all be sitting in the warm sunshine, wearing bathing suits and sunglasses, with our bodies glistening from sunscreen and coconut scented oils. The waves will be crashing along the shore while perfect strangers walk along the beach with wagons full of coconuts, straws and a machete to slice off the top of the fruit before passing us the refreshments for five dollars each! We are about to embark on an entire week of family laughter, smiles and the pure and utter joy of being able to spend time together without the constant interruption of work, telephone calls, Emails and the daily torture of ordinary life! And it's exactly what the doctor has ordered for me! The very same doctor that is going to slice into my body and remove the alien being that's taken root along the inside lining of my right lung, told me to enjoy myself while on vacation! But I'm not going to think about the C-word this week! This week is about spending time with my husband and all five of my children! Even though the entire family clan is also flying in for the reunion in Puerto Rico, they are not my focus. MY family is my focus! There's no such thing as being tired on a day like today! There's no such thing as hitting the snooze button on a day like today! It is here and we are all skipping out the front door as we continually call out to each other:

"Does everybody have their ID?"

"Did everyone get a phone charger?"

"Does everyone have their phone?"

A melody of "Yes's and Got-it's" sing out as we load the car and settle into our seats in the giant big man car. Even the dog has been tucked away under the watchful eye of the twin's best friend. The lights are off except for the front outside porch, the doors and windows are locked, and finally we are on our way as Albert backs the giant big man car out of the driveway.

"Who wants a breakfast sandwich?" My question is immediately met with four sounding 'YES's as I pass the English muffin, egg, cheese and bacon sandwiches around the car. Last night one of the last things I did was to pack a cooler of drinks, mixed nuts, and chips and premade breakfast sandwiches for this morning. And just before we skipped out the front door, I had microwaved the sandwiches, wrapped them in foil and thrown them into a large canvas tote bag.

After devouring my own breakfast sandwich I could feel my body beginning to settle into my seat. My belly was full and the inside of the giant big man vehicle was so warm and so quiet. I leaned my head back onto the top of my seat, closed my eyes, and inhaled so deeply that I must have forced myself to slip into a deep and incredibly warm sleep. My eyes remained clamped shut as I felt the very core of my soul strolling along the crisp white sands of Culebra Island. The beach was completely deserted as my eyes looked far to the left and back around the lengthy horseshoe shaped shoreline, across to the right and far out in front of the spot at which I stood where the hook of the land seemed to kiss the very edge of the rising sun. It was as if I was standing at the very center of the entire world which was a perfect circle of land that just missed touching its two ends back together. In the middle of that opening of the nearly round beach was where the sunlight entered into the world of Culebra and in fact the sunlight was really the only thing powerful enough to enter into that world within the moment that I was standing there. The remoteness of the island made it unreachable by any other being and I was so blessed that I was able to stand there and enjoy such beauty of this earth.

The waves were so soft and gentle that they barely made a sound as they floated across the wet edge of the sands before sliding back into the immense body of the ocean. I could hear the scratching of the sand beneath my feet as I strolled toward the water. The wind was far off in the distance and beyond the boundary of land that protects the shore. The trees along the upper edge of the shoreline remained completely still except for the very top of their branches. Amongst the crisp fallen leaves and weed that grew in clumps amongst the underside of the trees I could hear the sudden scatterings of tiny lizards; cousins to the humungous iguanas that lurk amongst the shadows throughout the island of Puerto Rico. If not for the sudden skitterings of tiny lizards, soft waves and my own footsteps, the beach would be completely silent.

Slowly I stepped into the warm ocean. The water embraced my body like a long lost relative that's just come home after years of having vanished from the world. Not like the hug of a friend that you frequently spend time with. Not a hug that's nothing more than a full body hand shake. This embrace was the kind of hug that continues as the person clinging to you breathes and maybe for a moment begins to tear up because they are so incredibly happy to be able to touch you once again. And as the warm water off the shore of Culebra continued to embrace my entire body, I continued to walk deeper and deeper into it. The gentle surface of the ocean was just underneath my jawline as I closed my eyes and began to lean backwards and into the deepness of the ocean. I took a long deep breath in and just completely and utterly relaxed as my torso slowly rose to the swirls of current along the very top of the waves. I was floating. I was floating with my arms stretched out to my sides along the very surface of the rocking bosom of the ocean. Like a child that rests atop its mother's chest and cries, I felt my body rise and fall with the very breathing of the vast deep ocean along the shoreline of the tiny deserted island off the coast of Puerto Rico. And nothing else seemed to matter. Nothing else seemed to be important. The only thing that I felt at that moment of such an immensely warm and heaving embrace was complete and utter reliance.

"We're here!" The giant big man car suddenly jerked with an explosive screech as Albert pulled into the long term parking lot at the Manchester airport.

"Oh my God, I can't believe we're here!" One of the twins was already scampering from the car and digging through the back for her carry-on suitcase.

"Wow. That's went by so fast." I was smiling as I looked at

Albert.

"Have a nice nap?" He's irritated. I'm sure it wasn't exactly pleasant being the only person awake and responsible for the driving while the entire car slept and snored through the darkness in the wee hours of the morning.

"Sorry." Why am I apologizing? Didn't I make you a breakfast sandwich? That's more than enough fair and even trading for a one hour nap on the way to the airport.

"Everybody get your bags out!" He's barking orders at all of us as we stand there already holding onto our bags. He's the only one that hasn't gotten his bag from the back of the car. He's the only one that isn't bouncing up and down with excitement and he's the only one that seems to have a bad attitude. This is the drive into Boston all over again! Why does he always have to stress? I really do believe that I'm the only one on the entire planet that has the right to be stressed right now and it pisses me off every single time I witness anybody else getting agitated and more often than not that 'anybody else' seems to always be Albert! Really?!!!

"Let's go." I immediately spin on my heels away from Albert and start the short trek across the parking area to the entrance. A small cluster of people are scrambling ahead of us to get into the building and up to the airline counter first. There are two uniformed men along the sidewalk that are checking baggage in for other people, which I would just never be able to trust. How can those men assure me that my bags are not going to get lost and are actually going to find their way to the correct airplane and make the journey with me to the island of Puerto Rico? They can't. I don't understand the system or if they even have one and without that information I just will never trust it. I have a carry-on bag and a giant suitcase that I am checking, directly at the desk where I can see it disappear through the hole in the wall that has a curtain of rubber flaps hanging across the front of it.

"Hello, how are you this morning?" I'm smiling as I hand the lady behind the counter all of our tickets and Albert hoists the large suitcase onto the side-counter scale contraption. The suitcase can't weigh more than forty pounds or we will be forced to pull contents from within it and shove them into our carry-ons, which cannot weigh more than twenty-two pounds each.

"We have a problem." The lady behind the counter has

159

stopped smiling.

"Oh no. Does it weigh too much?" I knew it! I knew it when I told Albert that we didn't need to pack snorkeling gear last night. They always have those things for rent at the beaches for a lousy five bucks or so; why on earth do we need to pack that crap and struggle with more weight in the suitcase all the way from New Hampshire to Puerto Rico when we can rent the stuff right there for such a small amount of money? And his logic is, 'why would I rent what I already own?' Seriously?

"No. Not at all."

"Oh good! Then what's the problem?" I'm smiling as I notice that the suitcase only weighs thirty-eight pounds. Thank goodness I don't have to rummage through and pull out items heavy enough to lower the weight of the freaking thing! But then again the only one that would have been impacted would have been Albert because I would have totally made him march through the airport carrying all of the snorkeling gear! Those are the items that potentially added the extra weight. It certainly couldn't have been my five pair of sandals!

"Your flight's been cancelled."

Chapter 31

I can't stop crying!

I'm quite literally sobbing and quivering as I struggle to wipe the tears so I can focus on the highway and signs that point me in the right direction to get back home. It's still dark out and there's a bit of fog that is wafting across the highway which seems to twist and turn with the bending branches of tall trees that sway to the left and right along both sides of the road. Thomas is sitting in the front passenger seat and he is quietly looking out the window. The twins are in the back seat and they are screaming and demanding that this not be happening to us right now! They are crying out loud as they swear for revenge against the person responsible for causing this tragedy and they don't even know who that person is. None of us do. We can't understand what has just happened and why we are being punished. We are supposed to be on an airplane right now! We are supposed to be just a few short hours away from the delicious food and warm beaches! Why is this happening to us?!

And Albert is gone. He got on a plane. He was the only person that was able to get onto another flight and actually make it to our destination on time. There was only one stinking single seat on the only other flight going to Puerto Rico today and he was the only logical choice for taking that one single seat. Our other two children that don't live at home are both flying in from other airports and they both need to be picked up from the airport late this evening. Who's going to do the picking up if none of us are there? Who's going to get the rental car? Who's going to drive to the rented condo to meet the owner, pay the rest of the rental money, and get the key? Who's going to drive back to the airport hours after that to get our two children? And that condo is a mere forty minutes from the airport! Who's going to figure out how to do all of that and how to find their way to the condo, back to the airport and back to the condo again and again? Not me! I don't think I'd be able to figure out all of that without knowing a single lick of Spanish. Albert's WAY better at all of that stuff and he knows the language! He's the only one that gets to go.

The rest of us have been put on hold. On hold for an entire day. On hold because of some horrific mechanical issue that erupted on the airplane that we were all supposed to be sitting in at this very moment. The silver lining of course being that we are all safer because of the decision to cancel the flight, rather than endanger the lives of more than two hundred innocent people. Nonetheless we are not the least bit happy or relieved at having been put on hold for any reason whatsoever!

The red blinking light on the telephone has been pushed and we are sitting and waiting in limbo until the operator picks the other end of the telephone back up. And there's some stupid song from the eighties playing in the background, while we continue to wait and we are forced to listen to it! And the whole time we continue to wait for that voice to come across the line we continue to curse the name of the person who made the decision to cancel the flight, even though we still have no idea who that person really is. And it will be a while! That operator won't pick the phone back up for nearly another twenty-four hours and by that time the song that we hate will be forever bored through a hole in our pissed off, screaming and crying brains! We are on hold until tomorrow morning when we get to do it all over again at three thirty in the morning when we head back to the airport and pray to GOD that our flight doesn't get cancelled again! So for now we are just going to cry.

I have no words. I have nothing but emptiness and sadness. I'm sad for Albert going through the airport and two flights alone, having to figure out how to get there, get the car, find the condo, pick up our other children and then sit and wait for the rest of us to arrive tomorrow mid-morning. I'm sad for my two children that are going to be picked up at the airport in San Juan by ONLY Albert, later today and they have no idea what has happened to the rest of us. If I were Albert, I'd be buying a big giant bottle of rum and some mango juice the second I picked them up and got them delivered to the condo!

I'm sad for my children in the back seat that are completely sobbing as their bodies heave back and forth with the swaying of the giant big man car as I jerk the steering wheel around the curves in the road. I'm sad for Thomas who is completely silent as he continues to stare out the front passenger window. And I'm positive that the three of my children that are with me are waiting for me to fix this. I'm positive that the crying and the silent staring will not stop until I figure out a way to save the day!

I need to save the day the way I did when they called me from school because they had forgotten their assignment and they needed me to drop everything and drive it across town. Or like the day I needed to find the glue to repair a handmade Christmas ornament that was dropped onto the tiled kitchen floor. Or like the time I needed to rush across town to the emergency room because the cut was just a bit too deep for a mere bandage. And they all looked at me and smiled because 'Mom fixed it.' But this time I have nothing. I cannot control a single bit of anything that is happening to us right now. There is nothing that I can fix, or glue or deliver to make this not have happened to the family. Even if I drive as fast as I can and scream through the doors of the emergency room begging for somebody to stop the bleeding it won't work! This can't be fixed! And I didn't see it coming. There is nothing that I could have possibly done differently to have made this not happen to us. So now I just have to make the best of it. I need to remember and realize that it's just a moment. It's a moment that crying will not fix. It's a moment that we will get through. Our lives are made up of many millions of tiny, confusing, sometimes big, happy or sad moments. The moments can impact us and they can cause us to react and sometimes we can even learn from those many moments. The moments are really only the adventures within our lives, they are not the definitions of them.

"Let's do this!" I'm not going to cry anymore. I look into the rear view mirror and see the sobbing faces of my two youngest children. Thomas has fallen asleep.

"What?" They are both shaking.

"Let's keep the bags in the car, drive straight to the salon for pedicures, pick up Chinese food, and go home to curl up in front of the television and watch movies!"

They both are still wiping away tears. For a moment there is nothing but silence in the giant big man vehicle. Finally one of them speaks: "Can we get our eyebrows done too?"

The twins and I immediately burst out laughing, which causes Thomas to wake up and viciously rub his eyes. "What's going on?"

"We're going to go get our toes done? Do you want to go also?"

"Nope. Just drop me off at home first and I'll go fishing." Quietly he rolled back into his seat and closed his eyes. The twins and I just continued to giggle as we headed back to the house to drop off Thomas. Somehow we would find a way to make the best of the situation and get through just one more day. Somehow we would just imagine ourselves in the warm waters off the shore of Culebra as we all just decide to swim.

Chapter 32

So the good news is that today's flight is direct! And the better news is that our flights weren't cancelled! I'm completely positive that I got zero sleep last night in anticipation of getting to the airport, parking the car, shuffling into the airport and getting onto the freaking airplane with three of my young adult children and without Albert's assistance. But I should be able to handle it! I traveled for years as a Regional Manager for a large Maine based retail company. I never had a helper back then and I made it to my destinations in one piece. AND back then there were no such things as GPS's. I had to get there using a map and driving through areas that I'd never in my life imagined I'd visit. And I did it. Today should be easier than that; but I still couldn't sleep last night.

"Where are the breakfast sandwiches?" One of the twins is yawning as she snickers from the back seat of the giant big man vehicle. We all chuckled and whole heartedly agreed that we were too nervous to eat anyway. We just wanted to get onto the plane!

By the time we got to the airport and approached the counter with our tickets in hand I was practically crying. I honestly don't know how I'm going to react if that lady behind the counter tells me that our flight has been cancelled. I am positive that I'm going to completely break down into a bursting river of tears if she says that. It's either that or I'm going over the top of the counter with my twins and youngest son joining me and we will all four go completely ham on her ass!

"Good morning." I'm faking a smile as I intently study the woman behind the counter's face. Is she going to drop her smile just like the lady from yesterday did? Is she going to pretend that everything is okay just before ripping the rug out from underneath us all once again? I don't think I can handle it if she does. I NEED to get onto the plane today! No delays and no unforeseen circumstances PLEASE! The lady behind the counter is staring at her computer screen as she flips through ticket after ticket. She's not asking us any questions. Why isn't she asking us any questions? She's tapping the keys on her computer and she's pursing her lips and crossing her brows. What the hell is she doing anyway? Why the hell isn't she saying anything? I'm starting to sweat! It's getting progressively hotter and hotter in here and I can't for the life of me understand who the hell is cranking the heat up when it is actually quite pleasant outside! Is there somebody that has just shown up for their shift at the airport and they recently moved here from the Equator? They just plopped themselves down at their desk and they suddenly decided that the entire building was too cold. They decided for themselves and the rest of us innocent customers that we would be much more comfortable if the dry crisp airport air was suddenly cranked to a thick balmy ninety degrees. And as we the customers continue to stress in anticipation of just getting onto the freaking airplane, we now have the added benefit of dripping pools of sweat down our back, underneath our arms and under what is now a sopping wet mane of tangled hair on the back of our necks!

"Your flight is on time and you will want to head over to gate 3D." She's smiling.

And now I'm crying again; just like yesterday but for the opposite reason.

"Thank you!" All four of us screamed at the lady, snatched our tickets and began running through the airport. We looked like a scene from 'Home Alone' as we charged through the crowds, through the gated security checkpoint and onward to gate 3D! And as our luck would have it gate 3D is literally next to a breakfast, donut and coffee stand! The best part about overpaying for breakfast sandwiches at the airport is that you don't have to make them!

When the four of us are finally sitting on the plane we are finally drying our tears as we reminisce about yesterday morning over and over again. We are beyond excited and a bit satisfied that the airline has given us credit coupons for two-hundred dollars towards future flights because of the inconvenience of losing an entire day from our Puerto Rico vacation! It's not enough as far as I'm concerned but it's better than no apology. And it wasn't until the plane was actually in the air that I knew we were really going to make it to Puerto Rico!

It's the third time we have been there. The first time was when my oldest went to college there and we were so completely lost. Albert did a phenomenal job of getting us around the island. We saw so many amazing things; fish so brilliantly colored they looked like cartoons and sea urchins that walked across our palms when we plucked them from the ocean floor. I never knew that sea urchin legs are actually long and a deep burgundy-red color. I thought they were short stubby and green; the way they look when you find just the shells along the very edge of the beach.

And then I thought about the views. I can't wait to see the views again. Words cannot really describe the views of the entire island as you stand in the lookout tower at the top of the rainforest. We will be there so soon and I can't wait to just relax and take it all in, all over again, with my family! And all I have to do is close my eyes and in a blink I'll be on the beach!

If I can just fall asleep the time will disappear. Time will disappear and I will be there. I just need to sleep.

Chapter 33

As quick as I got there after falling asleep on the airplane, it was all over again and I was back home. I blinked and the entire week had flown by and we were driving back home from the airport. There were so many moments of sincere beauty with my family that I will carry with me always. There were so many unbelievably beautiful things as there always seems to be when we visit Puerto Rico. And the fact that this particular trip was a family reunion vacation, which included some of my many nieces, nephews, sister in-laws and brother in-laws made the trip just that much more important. And given the fact that I'm completely terrified of what lies in store for me in just two days, the moments that we shared in Puerto Rico seem even more important than they would have been before the discovery of the 'something's there'.

Thank God the family drama that always seems to accompany these reunion trips was not because of me nor about me! Not that it ever has been but I truly dread the idea of suddenly being thrust into a clamoring room full of pissed off relatives that are screaming at each other and demanding satisfaction for something that in the grand scheme of things is truly not all that important. Every single time we have gone on one of these trips there is some sort of explosion. Four years ago the explosion was between another two of the sister in-laws; different sister in-laws from the prior reunion explosion. Apparently one of them had commented that the other's adult children should have been able to attend the trip because they'd had the entire two years prior to it to save and prepare. That comment completely irritated the other and at that point it was on! The screaming match followed only to be shushed and redirected by the oldest brother of all of the seven siblings that attended. Fortunately I was the only person that missed the entire showdown! I was cooking dinner in the kitchen, while the rest of the family fought at the picnic tables outside. And I was okay with missing it although when the other family members laughed, mimicked and shared the details with me I sort of wished I'd seen it. But I saw the drama this time! And this time it was between Albert and one of his bratty younger brothers. This time I got to witness the entire episode. This time I stood there with my heart beating out of my chest, while Albert took control of the situation and demanded that the younger sibling show some sort of consideration for the rest of the family rather than running off on his own and refusing to spend the time together as everyone had originally planned. Why on earth would you even want to spend the money to fly a family of five to Puerto Rico and then just ignore, lie and maliciously intend to dampen spirits or exclude people from having a good time? Just so you can be standing there at the end of the week gloating that your family got to do something that the others didn't? Where is the joy in that? What do you gain by purposefully hurting other people? Or maybe that's how you thrive? Maybe that's the breath that keeps you living? Maybe that's the joy in YOUR life? So sad.

And there were two times in particular during the week that we spent in Puerto Rico that I actually for the first time realized that something is physically wrong with me. For the first time I noticed some alarming 'things' happening to my body that I'd never noticed before. And I wonder if I would have ignored them had I not known otherwise that something was already wrong? I wonder if I would have just assumed I was coming down with something, or getting old, or maybe had too many coconut and rum drinks the night before? One of the episodes was when we had decided to do some low-level hiking to the top of the rain forest. The hiking was really just walking up a paved path that winds up and up and up until you reach an incredibly tall, stone watch tower that sits at the very top of the forest. And once you climb up and into that tower and you look out over the edge of the tall stone structure, you can quite literally see the entire island and hundreds and hundreds of miles of open ocean, waves, boats and low lying clouds over water that is the bluest water I've ever seen. It is stunningly beautiful!

But the walk to the top of that mountain and to the top of the stone tower nearly killed me. And it's not like I'm a completely physically fit person but at the same time it's not like I'm not either. I'm five feet and ten inches tall and I weigh approximately one-hundred fifty-five pounds. When I was in school (many years ago though) I participated in basketball, softball, swimming, and cross-country track. And since those years I've been running around chasing after five children, working full-time on my feet for more than twelve hours a day, and attending every sporting event or band concert that my children participated in! So I'm sort of in shape. But I didn't feel like I've ever for a second even known what it was like to have any sort of physical stamina when I was struggling to walk to the top of that mountain. In fact I even struggled when we walked back down to where the cars were parked along the side of the winding paved roadway. My chest heaved. My body tingled. I felt like what I imagined to be a massive asthma attack even though I've only had a few minor bouts with asthma due to sitting too close to campfires. I couldn't breathe. And I couldn't wait for it to just be over. I needed to get my body off of that mountain, back to the car and into the cooler that sat in the way back of our car and held multiple bottles of ice cold water. My daughters were staring at me as I struggled with the hiking/walking. They'd never seen me have such a reaction to such a slight physical challenge. Suddenly I could tell that something was wrong with me. Suddenly I could tell that the tumors, which the surgeons had all told me about and showed to me, were really inside of me. Suddenly I realized that I was sick.

The second time that it happened we had gone to the Island of Culebra. We had to take a ferry over from the main island to get to the remote location. The beach was so beautiful! The sand was white and the water was jade and turquoise. I was thankful that along the edge of the beach, where the sand meets the forest, there were multiple food shacks. Local families cooked empanadas, chicken on sticks, lots of rice, and even the simplest of burgers and fries. The weather couldn't have been more perfect on that day. Every day in Puerto Rico the weather seems to be perfect and on that day it was even more perfect than usual. After a couple of hours of being in the sun, I found myself hiding from the harshness of the rays on my whiter than white skin and decided to just stand in the water with my Pina Colada and wide brimmed straw hat. One of my sister in-laws stood with me and we chatted about our kids and their successes. And the longer we stood there talking the deeper and deeper we were pulled into the water. Eventually I was standing neck deep in the lukewarm ocean of extreme saltiness when I once again realized that I was sick.

For my entire life I have swum in oceans, lakes, ponds and

swimming pools and have never had any issue with any sort of discomfort from the pressure of the water as it embraced every inch of my body. But on the particular day when we discovered the Island of Culebra I suddenly felt as if my chest were being pressed in from all directions and eventually the pressure was going to cause the complete destruction and probable implosion of my weakening heart. As I stood there chatting with my sister in-law I suddenly looked at her and said that I needed to get out of the water. She was so confused and immediately concerned. I had told her the story. I had told her about the tumors that are growing within the lining of my right lung. I had told her about my surgery and what they were going to have to do to my body to get the tumors out of me before they decide to replicate into another location thereby slowly killing my entire being.

"Are you okay?" She stared at me with horror.

"I feel like I'm having a heart attack. I need to get out of this water."

Quickly we moved toward the shore. And as soon as the water was below my waist I began to feel normal again. I turned to her and explained that I thought everything was fine and we both breathed a huge sigh of relief. It must have been the pressure of the water around my torso that caused the incredible pressure within my chest. It must have been a certain level of water or a certain depth that suddenly caused the horrific explosion within my ribcage. An explosion so incredible that I just knew I would not be able to continue breathing if I stayed underneath that certain depth or level of water for even a moment longer than I already had. Suddenly I knew I was sick, again.

But if it hadn't been for those two moments when I felt I truly had some physical limitations because of some sort of mysterious illness that I had never even known I had, until the Orthopedic Center stumbled upon it, I wouldn't have thought about the upcoming surgery. My week with my children, husband and all of the 'others' was near perfect! Even with the drama and bickering, a bit of a sunburn, and the pressure of keeping the entire group fed and entertained, all in all it was a wonderful week. Every day was an adventure full of laughter, smiles and the normal compromises that we have come to accept as a way of life with a large family. Every day I thought about how much I truly want to just move to Puerto Rico. Every day I imagined that I could open a small diner for tourists that are looking for a taste of home as they journey through the challenge of trying to recognize food as they are ordering it. Every day in Puerto Rico I looked to the future and dreamed for what perhaps will be reality at some point in my life. But before I knew it had happened the entire week was gone except for the final day. The final day had now arrived and the serene beauty of the island would very quickly be far behind me. It was on that final day that we decided to journey to a tourist destination that took us nearly two hours to get to. And it was not until that final day that I became anxious to just get on with things!

For our final day of vacation we went to what I can only describe as 'The Caves'. We had only heard of them and we had researched a bit on the internet and the photographs looked really stunning! Never in my entire life had I ever gone inside a cave of any sort and the pictures on the internet of these ones in particular seemed that they could be nothing but completely overwhelming! We were all excited and the two hour drive seemed like a mere blink of an eye and we were pulling into the parking lot.

There weren't that many people going to the caves on that particular day; my guess is that they must be quite a bit busier on weekends. As we all filed through the front doors of the welcome facility we were greeted by a "Cave-Person" who handed us all tiny radios with attached headphones. The Cave-Person explained that the tour was guided and in order to ensure that everybody could hear everything, they recommend that we all wear the one-way radio so we could enjoy all that the caves have to offer.

Next we all were directed to sit in a jeep-sort-of-train thing that followed along a very winding, corkscrew shaped path of pounded dirt through the jungle. We anxiously sat and held on tight as the jeep-train jerked, veered, and twisted along the path that seemed to sink deeper and deeper into the tall woods. The journey seemed longer than I would have imagined it needed to be. It felt like the caves should have literally been out the back door of the welcome facility but they weren't. The sky was disappearing as we continued to drive deeper and deeper into the jungle. There were flowers hiding amongst the thick green leaves of the draping canopy and they looked like pink explosions of huge sea urchins. The air became thicker and thicker as we continued to sink. And the darker and the deeper that the jungle became, the colder and colder atmosphere became. As happy as I was to embark on a journey beneath the very crust of the earth I suddenly felt an inner twinge of uncertainty and fear. Fear that I was about to enter into an unknown and hidden place. Fear that for some reason my stomach was beginning to churn and twist with every turn and twist of the path that we continued to rumble through. Where is this place? How much further do we need to twist and spiral, lower and lower into the deepness of the dark and thick jungle full of huge trees, draping vines and flowers that I don't recognize?

"Everybody out!" The driver of the train of jeeps suddenly slammed the contraptions into park and ordered us off of the ride.

And there it was, there it stood and there it breathed in the side of a massive hidden mountain of earth. The mouth of the cave was so enormous! And I could already see what resembled teeth, dripping from the upper side of the roof of the cave's mouth. And we were walking directly into it. We walked in a single line with our headphones on and our tiny radios turned to channel four. And the man that had driven us there was speaking to us and directing us to look above our heads, or over to the left, or the right, and to watch our steps because the rocks within the mouth were slippery. And blindly we all followed. We just listened and we just followed the direction that he gave us. And we don't know this man that led us into what could very well have been a monstrous mouth full of huge fangs that would slam shut the second our tiny beings tripped through the very edge of the opening but we listened to him anyway.

Suddenly it was so dark. And the air somehow became incredibly cold; as cold as the air back home can get even on a summer evening. I couldn't see a thing. I wanted to reach out and touch the side of the walls within the monstrous cave but I was too scared to reach away from my torso. I could hear water dripping and I was choking thick cold air deeply into my lungs as I struggle to keep up with the single line of tourists that I followed. My family was behind me and they were accepting that I must have been comfortable and knew where I was going even though I was completely terrified as I ventured into the unknown.

The deeper we crept through the twisting stone paths within the monstrous cave, the more I began to recognize my surroundings as an all too familiar scene. Something within this cave reminded me of a place I had been before. The darkness, the thickness of the air, the sound of dripping were all too familiar as I quietly and blindly continued to walk to the very back of the cave's throat. And the tour guide was still directing us and he was practically yelling as he told us all to hang onto the rope fence that bordered a giant black hole that he expected us to tiptoe past and hopefully not teeter over the edge and into, never to be found again as our bodies flailed and spun, falling deeper and deeper into a hole that undoubtedly has no exit or end. As I slowly ventured past the giant black hole I couldn't help but look down and into the vast space of nothing but blackness and it was then that I realized exactly where I was. And the terror of the sudden realization overwhelmed my very being and I immediately began to cry.

My tears were streaming down my face as I stared into the deeper and darker hole and suddenly I felt my body spinning out of control as once again I was falling. My arms were slapping and digging into the side of the earth, desperately trying to grab hold of any stone ledge, tree root or chunk of clay. And I knew it was the freaking Canterbury well, again. It was following me and had left the edge of the property that we loved and it had found its way to the massive caves of Puerto Rico! And when I tried to just peek into the deep dark hole, I once again accidentally stepped too far over the edge. Just the same as I did when I strolled along the edge of the farmhouse property years ago; I stumbled and now I was falling deeper and deeper into the darkness. As hard as I tried I could not grab ahold of the edge of the well and my struggle did nothing but cause my desperate body to sink deeper and deeper into the unending darkness. I could not see what was at the bottom of the huge dark hole and the little bit of light that the cave dwellers had installed for the tourists to barely see their way along the slippery stone path, were becoming dimmer and dimmer as I fell further and further into the hole and away from the very edge that I toppled over. I was screaming at the top of my lungs and I panicked as I twisted and tore through the sharp stone edges of what must have been the very throat at the back of the horrific monstrous mouth. I was screaming and I was crying out for somebody to save me! I needed somebody to help me! I needed to stop falling and flailing within the darkness that had completely enveloped my body, my thoughts, and my very soul which just continued to slip and slide away from the teeny flickering of light. And I couldn't face what was happening to me! I couldn't face that I was completely helpless and I couldn't stop myself from falling and falling, deeper and deeper into the darkness. And I couldn't stop myself from screaming over and over again: 'I don't want to fight! I cannot do it! I am losing the battle and I am going to be lost in the darkness of this treacherous cave for all eternity! Help me God! Somebody help me, PLEASE! Why is this happening?!'

"Are you okay?"

I was breathing so hard and I was completely frozen as I continued to look over the edge of that cliff within the monstrous cave. I had imagined the darkness to be nothing more than the very end of my existence. And as I turned to face that voice that called out to me, I found myself once again staring into my husband's eyes.

"Just keep moving." Gently he touched my arm.

And that was all it took for me to continue my journey through the monstrous caves in Puerto Rico. Just around the bend and away from the edge of the throat of the earth, we began to see the sunlight streaming through the entrance. And when we walked back out of the incredible mouth I began to feel the sudden warmth of the tropical air embracing my shivering body.

"Everybody out!" Albert jerked the car into park as we came to a stop. We were back home and had pulled into the driveway of our new house. The vacation was over.

Chapter 34

Oh my God, tomorrow is the day of my surgery and I'm completely and utterly terrified. I know that I have no choices here. I know that I need to get the growing alien being out of my body before it starts a colony full of identical beings which it somehow manages to procreate but I don't want to! I don't want to be doing this! I don't want to have this thing inside of me and I don't want to be in pain after they freaking cut it out of me either! I cannot win! I have to do this!

I can't stop thinking about that one little question! I can't shake it and I find myself once again screaming within my own mind and asking myself how did this happen in the first place? What did I do, because I'm sure it must have been something that I did to myself because if it was not because of something that I foolishly chose to do wouldn't everybody on the planet have the exact same thing as me? It's something that I did, something that I exposed myself to or something that I ingested. It's not genetics because my mother, father, sister or brother do not have the thing that I have inside of me. So what was it? What did I do? I need to figure it out and I need to make sure that none of my children repeat the same horrible mistake that I obviously made!

How could I have done this? How could I have done something that potentially will crush my husband and my five children? What was I thinking about when I did this to myself? And how am I ever going to ask for their forgiveness when they are watching me suffer with freaking cancer, knowing that it's for my own selfish reasons that it's happened anyway?

It must have been all the years of bartending in the mid-eighties, before I was even married and before I ever knew I was going to be a mother of five. Everybody smoked. I smoked. The air that we breathed was so thick that you couldn't even see through it to the other side of the room. It was like being in a giant gray cloud.

I'm really starting to think that it must have been the sandbox that my father built in the back yard. Where did those giant barrels of dirt come from that he poured into the wooden frame that he built?

Then again maybe it was the red M&M's that I used to dig through the package for, so I could eat them all before my little brother got his grimy hands on them?

I keep playing my entire life over and over in my head trying to figure out how I did this. Whatever it was it's my fault! I breathed it, I touched it or I ate it! I made the stupid decision and now I'm going to have to deal with the consequences of that stupid decision all because I had to make that one fatal choice. That one fatal and horrific choice that has caused pain and suffering for my entire family and I can't for the life of me figure out what the one thing was that I shouldn't have done! How could I have done this?!

Maybe I deserve it. Maybe I haven't been a good enough person all these years. I'm sure there are a lot of people that can't stand me and will more than likely celebrate when they hear that I have cancer. The people that I had to fire for one reason or another over the years are probably still bitter. They are going to be more than excited to hear that I'm going to be suffering. They'll all say I deserve it and they will believe that it's Karma. And maybe it is.

"How you doing?" The snake is hissing and flickering her tongue at me as she slowly slithers into my office.

"I'm fine." What the hell does she want? She'll be one of the ones celebrating if she hasn't already started. "I'm putting some final touches on the e-mail for you all, explaining who will be responsible for what while I'm out on my medical leave."

"Oh, okay. That sounds good." For some reason she sits in a chair across from my desk.

I stop typing and just look at her.

"I just want you to know that I'll be thinking about you, I hope everything goes well and if you need anything just let me know." I can see her tongue dancing around behind her teeth when she stops talking. I'm sure she desperately wants to point it at me as it snaps, hisses and flickers, while her eyes slowly begin to squint from across the room.

"Thank you." I'm completely struggling to see her as a human being. I know she doesn't care about what happens to me. I know she's just putting on a show and for some reason trying to put herself in a better light with me but it's not going to work.

She's nothing more than a serpent that will begin to devour more and more prey the second I leave the store today. I don't trust her and I don't believe her.

With that she left and I quickly finished a few more last minute 'things' before shutting down my computer and locking the door to my office.

Chapter 35

My mother arrived at my new house just shortly after dinner.

"You okay?" Slowly she sipped on a small glass of wine from across the living room. She looks worried.

"I'm okay. Just want to get it over with." I feel sick. I have never been as scared as I am right now. I've had surgeries but never anything like this one. I can't get my head around how on earth they will manage to peel the lining from around my lung and therefore remove the tumors that are boring down on the nerves that run underneath my armpit. How are they possibly going to manage to get that done without sawing my freaking torso in half? I don't get it!

Two of my daughters are still here with me and have been here since returning from our vacation. They took extra time off from their jobs and they don't have classes this time of year. My oldest son went back home to Maine and my oldest daughter went back home to Florida.

"How are you feeling Mom?" One of the twins asked the question and they both are looking at me from across the room and are flipping through channels trying to find a show that they don't get on their limited plan of cable channels at the dorm.

"I'm fine." I'm not fine though. I'm freaking out! Why did I even let them come? I'm pretty sure I asked them to. Why would I have done that to them? Isn't it enough that I caused whatever I'm about to go through; I had to selfishly invite them to stand beside me while I do it? For what? Why did I do that to them?

My two daughters, mother, Albert and I are getting up and leaving by three o'clock in the morning. I have to be at the hospital in Boston by five o'clock. And I can't eat anything or drink anything after midnight.

I don't want to go. I feel empty. And I'm scared. What's going to happen if I die? Oh my God, how is it that I can even say that word? Is this how it's going to all end for me? Is this the last day of my actual life? Is this the last time I'm going to see my family? What am I supposed to say to them other than 'I love you'??

Can they tell that this is what I'm thinking? None of us are even talking. We're quietly sitting in the living room and now we're watching some stupid comedy movie that the twins found on television. I don't know the name of it and I don't know who's acting in it and I don't even freaking care right now! I can hear the noise from the movie and I'm staring at the television but I'm not registering any of it whatsoever. I just want to go to sleep so we can wake up, drive to the hospital and be done with all of this.

I need to stop thinking. I need to be completely out of time and have nothing more to think about and nothing more to question and no more opportunity to beat myself up and blame myself for the stress and discomfort that I'm causing everybody by getting stuck with the freaking cancer growing inside of my body! I should just go to bed. I should just run upstairs and fly across the room and into my bed, pull up the covers and slam my head down on the pillow. If I just go to sleep, it will be time to go to the hospital. Once I'm at the hospital, I won't be able to think because the nurses and doctors will just keep asking me questions over and over again!

I just need to sleep.

Chapter 36

"Shit. It just got real."

I'm sitting in a hospital gown, in a bed that is more than freaking cold and all I really want right now is for a nurse to come in and give me some sort of drug of some sort so I can just calm the fuck down! Where the hell are all the nurses anyway? Aren't there like ten thousand nurses that work here?

We arrived at the hospital exactly on time and I was shocked when we entered the registration waiting room. There must have been a hundred people with family members, all waiting to be registered so they too could sit in a gown, in a freezing cold bed, as they wait for their turn in an operating room.

The twins were already pissed off. They had for some reason decided to just NOT go to bed last evening; figuring that it would be easier than waking up at three o'clock in the morning. When three o'clock came they quietly asked me if they could just not go with me to Boston after all. They were too tired and asked if 'Dad can just call us when it's over.' And when that question presented itself to me I dove head first into a burning pit of rage. When what's over? When I'm dead? Is that what they mean with that question because it is a very real possibility that I can just die on the table and will never see them or anybody else in my family or in my life for that matter ever again! So of course I yelled at them and now am sitting here freezing in a hospital bed, again feeling like the most selfish person on the planet. What the hell is wrong with me anyway? Why am I doing this to them? Why didn't I just let them go to bed and get some rest? I'm the meanest mother in the world. Now I have the added burden of feeling not only guilty for getting cancer, but now I am also guilty of forcing my daughters to accompany me to the hospital.

"Would you like a warm blanket?" The door to my room opened with a massive 'swoosh' as a male nurse danced into the room. I already love him!

"God YES!"

"Chilly?"

"Yes. Please."

I began to feel a bit warmer with my wonderful blanket even though the room remained bitter and cold. My amazing nurse danced around the room and made sure that all of my 'stuff' was in order, that my personal belongings were in a clearly labeled plastic bag, and that my family took any valuables away from me such as my cell phone or money. And just as he became satisfied with the organization of my stuff, he spun around and politely asked my two daughters, Albert and my mother to exit. Something about putting in an arterial line/IV of some sort. And I wasn't sure why he needed to clear the room until I looked at the aftermath. My bed was completely doused with enough blood that a passerby would have most assuredly assumed a massacre had just taken place.

"Wow."

"I know. Let me clean up the evidence of murder before your family comes back in." Both of us chuckled as my nurse quickly peeled the warm blanket and top sheet from my crimson bed.

When my mother re-entered the room she said she didn't understand why the nurse hadn't allowed her (a retired nurse) to stay. I told her of the massacre and she calmly exclaimed that he didn't know what he was doing and that was why he had requested that the room be cleared. Both of us laughed out loud and I quickly realized that everything was funny to me. Time around me seemed to be crawling with the uncertainty of an infant that slowly rocks back and forth before placing one of its tiny little hands out in front of itself, thereby eventually moving forward at a glacier's pace. Once that first tiny little hand feels a speck of confidence, the infant rocks back and forth again and perhaps grunts little baby noises as drool slowly but most assuredly begins to form in a tiny puddle of slime beneath the rocking baby's smiling face. Eventually the second tiny little hand will attempt the same feat and the baby will continue to advance across the room. And that's me right now. A baby that is crawling in slow motion on a fast track to nowhere.

"What time are you supposed to be in surgery?" My mother is horribly nervous. She doesn't know what to say or what to talk about. She's about to watch her daughter be rolled away from her and into a room full of uncertainty and horribly dangerous circumstances. She doesn't want me to go into the room but she knows that I have to and she knows that she can't help me through it. She can only be there to tell me that she loves me and that it is going to be okay even though she doesn't know if it will. She's on the verge of bursting into a raging river of tears and wailing and her lips are quivering every time she speaks.

"Seven-thirty."

"They'll probably take you around seven o'clock then. Almost time." She's trying to smile as she pats my shoulder.

"Good morning!" The door to my room opens again but this time it's not the male nurse that I love.

"Good morning." I have no idea who I'm talking to right now.

"I'm Doctor Jaquelvickson and I'm your anesthesiologist." He's smiling as he reaches out an extremely clean looking hand and shakes mine.

"Hello." What the hell did he say his name is? I wonder where he's from. He looks to be of Indian decent. Indian meaning that he's from India and not a Native American.

"Do you know why you are here?"

"Yes."

"Can you tell me?"

"I'm having the pleura lining around my right lung removed." It's hard to even say. When I say the sentence the words just sort of get stuck in my mouth. They just don't flow. Some words just flow naturally, like 'gorgonzola cheese' or 'happy birthday' or 'I love you', but not 'I'm having the pleura lining around my right lung removed.' It feels like I'm trying to say a tongue twister and I still haven't truly figured out what a pleura lining even is!

"When is your birthday?"

More questions.

"What is your name?" I answered.

"What are you allergic to?" This question took me a bit longer to answer because for some reason I'm one of those people that is allergic to like twenty different types of medicines, vaccinations or pain killers.

"Okay. I'm going to take good care of you!" He's smiling. "I'll see you in there." And just like that he was gone again.

"Almost time." My mother is tearing up now. I can't look at her. Albert and the girls have gone to the cafeteria to get some breakfast. They said they'd be back before they wheel me down the hall but I have no confidence whatsoever that they will be back in time to say 'it's going to be okay' or 'you'll be fine.' And I'm not sure they'd say anything at all. I'm not sure what to expect from anybody other than my mother right now; she hasn't left my side. She keeps telling me that it's going to be just fine.

"Good morning." Who the hell is that? Another stranger has entered the room. "I'm Mary. I'm going to be taking care of you when you come out of surgery. I'm your recovery nurse."

"Hello." I'm smiling as she clicks a pen and begins to write something on the chart sitting on a sort of swing-arm-skinny desk thing next to my bed.

"Can you tell me why you're here today?" Again with the questions.

"I'm having the pleura lining thing that's around my lung cut out." I'm still stumbling with the words.

"Which lung?'

"Right."

"Okay, which one?"

"The RIGHT." I'm laughing at myself.

"Correct." Okay, she's a bit of a wise-ass.

"What is your birthday?" The same series of questions is asked all over again and we end with the nice nurse named Mary telling me that she's going to take great care of me and she'll get my family when I'm ready for them to visit.

"What time is it now?" I'm looking at my mother.

"Good morning!" An entire group of people have just entered the room and the person at the head of the crowd is my surgeon! He's here!!! He's the one that is going to save me! He's the one that has the knowledge, the skill and the power to rip the alien being from within my chest, throw it against the wall while it screams for help, charge over to it and just completely stomp it into a pulverized pile of pulsating alien being bloody flesh!

"HI!" I'm sitting straight up in my bed. I'm super excited that my surgeon is here! He's the only one that has ever given me a plan. He's the only one that knows exactly what to do. He's so confident and his demeanor is nothing but smooth! And besides all of that he is just wicked freaking smart!

Casually he took me through the steps of what he's still planning to do with my body once I'm under his knife. He spoke with both me and my mother about deflating my lung and removing the membranous lining that encases it. He said there was a chance that he would find 'more stuff' once he was in there and some decisions would be made within the moments of discovery but he would make sure to take great care of me. And I believed every word that he said to me and continued to nod my head throughout his speech. Then he pulled out a black felt tip marker and he wrote the words, 'CORRECT SIDE' across my arm.

"I'll see you in there." He winked and just like that Doctor Smooth exited my room with his entourage.

"I like him." My mother seemed to be relaxing just a bit with the information she'd received from the surgeon.

"Good morning!" Another person entered the room and I suddenly felt as if time was beginning to move very quickly. "I'm Scotty and I'm one of the nurses that will be in the operating room. Can you tell me why you're here today?"

"Yes." Her name is Scotty? I wonder if it's a nickname or if her last name is Scott. Maybe her real name is Ripley? She sort of looks like Ripley from the movie Alien, except her hair is lighter.

She's staring at me. I'm starting to giggle and I can't help but want to just mess with this woman. I've already answered the entire series of questions a number of times and am beginning to just want to entertain myself. I want to laugh out loud at the face staring back at me and I'm wondering if I'm actually going to fail the test she's about to deliver. She needs to ask the questions and she's probably got a million things to do. I'm sure she's not seeing any humor in me right now which is making me want to laugh even more and more.

"So, what are we going to be doing with you today?" She's remaining professional.

"You're going to be removing an alien being from my chest otherwise I will surely fall back onto a table screaming, as it explodes out of my rib cage and runs across the room before laying eggs in every room in the hospital, which will ultimately amount to more and more alien beings that will eventually take over the planet."

She's just staring at me while my mother giggles from the corner of the room.

She's not saying anything.

Still staring.

"You're removing the pleura lining from around my right lung." I'm trying to behave because I can see that this nurse just isn't going to have any of this.

She politely continued to ask the same questions that everybody else just did and I politely answered them all correctly. "I'm going to have the anesthesiologist's assistant come in and she's going to give you something to really relax you before we take you down the hall. Now would be the time for your family to give hugs and kisses."

Of course it is. "They're not here yet. They went to get breakfast."

"Well they have a few minutes before she comes in." And then she was gone. And then I started to panic.

First of all, where is my freaking family? Why couldn't they just wait and eat when I was having the surgery? They are going to have about five hours to kill while I'm under the knife. Why aren't they here? Do they even care about what is happening? Is the fact that they are tired and want a freaking blueberry muffin more important than holding my hand and telling me that I'm going to be okay before I embark on the scariest five hour adventure of my entire life? They don't care! They don't care at all! How is it possible that I'm a married for thirty years, mother of five and as I'm about to have surgery for freaking cancer I can't help but feel completely helpless, small, and absolutely alone!

"How's it going?" The door swung open again with another loud swoosh and suddenly Albert and the twins were standing there smiling.

"Oh, you're here?"

"What do you mean? Is everything okay?" One of the twins looks confused and concerned that they had just done something wrong, which of course in my mind they had but I wasn't going to say anything beyond the passively aggressive statement that I'd just made.

"They're coming in to take me to surgery any minute now. I just figured you weren't going to make it back in time." Okay, maybe I'll say something.

"In time for what?" Albert looks irritated with me.

They don't get it. They've never been through this, they've never even had a minor surgery and they aren't taking this seriously. They all collectively believe that everything is always going to be okay. And I guess that's a good thing. I guess I would certainly rather they think that than always the worst. I don't really know what I'm expecting from them right now. I don't think there's anything they can say or do that I will view as the perfect action or response.

"In time to give me a hug or something. You know...tell me it's going to be okay...tell me you love me." I can hear my voice quivering and I am suddenly beyond overwhelmed and completely terrified. I need to get the hell out of here. I don't want to do this! I'm scared! Somebody please help me and tell me that it's going to be okay! What will happen if I yank these things out of my arm and I just run for the door? They can't stop me, I don't think! They can't make me do this! It's my body isn't it? It's my life, right? I can leave! I'm leaving!!!

"How we doing?" Another complete stranger is in the room now. She's got a big smile on her face and she's holding a large syringe full of what appears to be milk. What does she actually think she's going to do with that?! And she better not ask me anymore questions because I am completely DONE! I'm not doing this! I'm leaving and all of these people with clipboards, questions, smiles and syringes full of milk need to take a step back and away from the freaking door!

"Fine." My voice is a quivering mess and I can feel the tears as they begin to pour down my face.

"I see I'm here just in time. You'll feel better in a second. Family!" She turns around and looks at the shocked faces of my two youngest children, my husband of thirty years, and my mother who has also crumbled into a sobbing pile of flesh; just like me.

"Okay." I leaned back my head and started to smile. I don't know what the milk actually was but I was glad she put it directly into the line in my arm.

I blinked my eyes and struggled to focus on my husband's face as he leaned over the bed and told me that he loved me and that everything was going to be okay.

Chapter 37

"Jane?"

I can't focus. Who's talking to me?

"Jane? Jane, how are you doing?"

I can't talk. Please don't wake me up. Please just let me keep sleeping. I don't want to open my eyes. I don't want to talk to you right now. Just let me sleep, please.

"Jane?"

Jesus Christ, she's not going to go away. "What?"

"Are you okay?"

No, now leave me alone. "Yes."

"Your family is here."

Tell them I'm sleeping. "Okay."

"Hi." Albert's still standing over me. Has he been there for long? Have they taken me into surgery yet? When are they taking me? Why don't they just move things along so we can get this over with already? What the hell??

"Hi."

"How are you feeling?" He looks so serious.

"Okay."

"She's going to be pretty groggy for a while. We'll move her up to her room now that she's waking up. Should be about an hour if you need to go get some dinner and then meet us in room 'four-forty-four."

"Okay. Come on guys!" Albert starts to spin around and I realize that the twins and my mother are standing behind him. This is a different room. There are things all around my bed that weren't there before. There's lots of beeping and clicking and tubes and lines all over my freaking body. There are computer screens in every direction that I turn my head. Where the hell am I? Did they do it already? They must have done it! What did they do? How did it go? Am I going to be okay? Did I make it? Is it over? My head is completely flooded with questions that I can't seem to get out of my head and through my mouth so somebody can tell me what's going on!

I'm slipping. I'm slipping back into the darkness! I can't

form any words and I can't seem to open my eyes enough to really focus beyond what is immediately around me. Where the hell am I and why is it getting so dark in here? Am I falling backwards? What are all the noises I keep hearing and how am I going to keep myself from sinking deeper and deeper into this darkness that is suddenly draping itself over the crisp and sterile whiteness of the room that we are all in? I'm falling! I'm definitely falling!!!

ALBERT! Where the hell did you go? Can't you see that I'm slipping back into the horrific darkness again? I must be falling into the well along the edge of the Canterbury property again! I need you to lean down and grab hold of the back of my neck or my mane of hair and just yank me back up! Don't let me fall back into this horrific stench of a well, full of nothing more than rotten corpses of tiny unfortunate animals that have slipped through the old boards that used to cover the entrance to the God forsaken well! It smells in here! It smells of putrid rotten corpses! And the corpses are floating just beneath my feet as I struggle to cling to the sides of the mud encased walls of filth, roots and chunks of clay. I can hear the rats and they're gnashing at my feet, hoping that I just slip deeper and deeper and then they'll be upon me. I'm slipping Albert! I can't pull myself back out! ALBERT! Where the hell are you? Where are you going?!

"Let's go get some dinner guys." He's spinning away from me and he's just going to walk away as I continue to fall deeper and deeper into the Canterbury well.

With every ounce of my energy I pushed my back against the filth of the well and reached as high above my head as my body would allow. I pressed my feet into the sides and I took in a giant life cleansing breath of the hot rancid air that filled the stench of that God forsaken well and I leaned forward and upward with everything that I had left! I could feel my body struggling to rise up towards the entrance. I could feel some movement of my torso and my legs as I pushed and pulled with all of my might. Suddenly I was moving ever so slightly as my feet slipped and twisted over the greasiness of the muddy walls. I was moving towards the top of the well. I was going to make it if I could just keep pushing and yanking and pulling my body up and out of that horrific dark rancid well. Slowly but assuredly I could feel my arm rising up from within and hitting the coolness of the breeze that quietly blew just above the very edge of the old rotten well. And I could see Albert standing there. He still stood above me as he spoke to my twins and my mother. With a sudden thrust of energy I reached out and grabbed for Albert's arm with all of my strength just as he turned away from me! I could feel the coolness of his skin underneath my filthy fingers that are completely covered with the sticky stench of the well. I can feel his skin just enough that if I curl my fingers inward, I might just be able to get the tips of my fingers around the side of his wrist! There it is! I can feel him! I have him!

And just as I grabbed hold of his arm he seemed startled. He jumped a little bit and snapped his head around and leaned down over my bed. His eyes were blood shot and he looked as exhausted as I felt. I struggled to breathe the coolness of the crisp air that seemed to blow through the sterile hospital room. And as soon as I gulped in that beautiful air I somehow managed to push it back out and through my lungs. I somehow managed to speak to my husband as I held onto his arm as tightly as I could.

"Please don't leave me."

Chapter 38

I remember the last time I saw my grandfather alive. He was living in a nursing home facility; only having been moved there when my poor grandmother had come to the realization that she could no longer provide the care that my grandfather needed. He was old. He was nearly ninety years old and he had Alzheimer's. He had always been a very proud man and was well thought of throughout the community. And when he became ill he started to do strange things and tasked my grandmother to the point that I'm positive he would have been so embarrassed of his own actions if he'd been able to realize what they were.

On the final day when I visited him he sat in front of a large window in the shared community room of the nursing home. And he looked so tiny and frail as he sat there with the brilliance of the sun shining through the grand window that served as his backdrop. And when I approached him he just stared at me. I remember my Gram saying to him, "Gar! Lynnie is here to see you."

My family had always called me by my middle name as long as I can remember. I guess I was just too cute for the planeness of 'Jane'. We all called my grandfather 'Gar' and I'm sure it was because my older sister couldn't pronounce Grandpa. So he was Gar and I was Lynnie.

"Oh?" He turned to look at me. When our eyes met and I smiled at him and it was then that I realized that I was looking at nothing more than blank thoughts and curiosities about who this young girl that stood before him was. He smiled but he was just being polite. He didn't know who I was and it was at that final moment that I saw him before his death when I realized what it meant to have the disease that he had. He was lost. Lost within a world that he didn't recognize or recollect. Lost within the darkness of a dark, deep, and lonely well. Lost as he floated amongst massive swells of a vast ocean. Lost within the darker than dark and dangerous forest. And he didn't know what to say to me. He didn't know how to react. He didn't know what to do when my grandmother told him my name after more than thirty years of knowing me. And he had always been the love of my life as well as all of my siblings and cousins lives. He had always been the kind of grandfather that LOVED his grandchildren and children. In all of the pictures that I look back on there isn't a single one of my grandfather in which he is not holding a child, grandchild or great-grandchild. He loved us. He lived for us. And he had lost us. He didn't know where we were nor why we were gone. We had all collectively just disappeared. And I wonder if the shenanigans of his actions were desperate attempts to find the ones that were lost. I wonder if he was desperately flailing out of control because the frustration of being so lost had finally erupted on the days that he tasked my grandmother the very most.

I didn't know what to say when I realized that he no longer knew who I was. I was frozen in time as I watched the blank expression on Gar's face spread across his smile and along the lines above his eyes. He was stuck in the darkness and because he was stuck, I began to also become stuck. I had no words. And after a few moments or so of staring blankly into my eyes he turned toward my grandmother and he looked into her eyes for some shred of direction for what he was supposed to do with the adult child that sat before him. The entire room was nothing more than the complete and utter sound of silence.

I watched as I sat and I knew not what to do with the scene that was bestowed upon me. As my grandfather gently turned his head and looked deeply into my grandmother's eyes it became clear. And it was then and only then that I realized what his world had become and what it truly had always been. His world had one meaning and that meaning was screaming loudly through the entire building as we sat in front of the larger than life windows behind my grandfather. The volume of that meaning was so incredibly loud as it raced from the meeting room, down the long gray hall that had only dim lights from fixtures that were installed when the building itself had been built more than fifty years prior. Down the narrow stairwells that had thick metal pipes for handrails and smelled of tomato sauce and urine, the meaning continued to run. It ran and it ran until it reached the ground level of the brick nursing home and then suddenly it burst through the double swinging doors! Out and into the parking lot it ran until it finally stopped, collapsed to its knees, leaned back and stared high up to the heavens and bellowed out what the meaning really is and has always only been! It screamed the only word that had and will always summarize my grandfather's life.

"LOVE!!!"

He loved her. Gar was so incredibly in love with my grandmother that she was the one and only thing, person, and possibility for his mind to still connect with the real world. She was all that he had left. And the look on his face when he turned to her and smiled, I will hold with me for my entire life. I watched as the confused expression and half-witted smile on my grandfather's face, completely melted and morphed into the gentlest of emotions I've ever witnessed. He slowly tipped his head to the right and he sighed through the most loving smile I'll ever see. And it happened when he saw her. It happened when he realized that she was there. And as my grandfather realized that the love of his life was still with him, he reached his hand out and he quietly and tenderly grabbed her arm. And I imagine that the words trapped within his mind as he smiled at the love of his life were the same as the words that I spoke to my husband on the day of my surgery:

"Please don't leave me."

Chapter 39

Everybody went home.

I had visitors every single day. But every single day they all continued to go home while I sat in the hospital recovering, sleeping, and walking.

My family went home on the actual day of my surgery as soon as I had been moved into an actual room. And it would be five more days until I'd be allowed to go home. And the days were all incredibly long even though I slept through nearly half of them. Albert came to visit every single day. Sometimes he brought one of his brothers along with him. And the whole while I was in the hospital, my body was being taken care of by some of the most incredible people I've ever met. Nurses that were so incredibly sensitive and so incredibly educated; they knew when and what I needed before it even happened. They never made me wait to take pain medicine, they let me order food whenever I felt I was hungry, and they FORCED me to get out of bed and keep walking down the halls, around the corners, back through the main desk area of the floor and into my room again; over and over and over they kept me moving. And initially I was irritated with them but as I began to actually feel like I was breathing again, I appreciated it. These nurses helped me begin my recovery.

There was one particular night that I really challenged this poor young girl that was taking care of me. I didn't mean to but I did and it was all because I simply don't like having a catheter in. I had kept the catheter in for two days but felt I had graduated to the point that I could make it into and out of the bathroom on my own, so no longer needed the horrific sensation that something is digging into the side of my freaking urethra. I requested that it be removed not realizing just how many times that would mean I would have to hoist my incredibly sore, battered, sliced up body into and out of the bed to go pee. Apparently when you are on a solid drip you pee a lot! There I was at three o'clock in the morning and of course I needed to go pee. I called the little girl in that was helping me through that particular night; she wasn't little as in a tiny person but she seemed little to me because I felt so much older than her. She maneuvered my IV bag, multiple tubes, plugs and just lots and lots of STUFF so I could make my way across the rather large and private room to my large and private bathroom. I was tired. I was so tired and so sore that I truly thought I must be completely insane for having them remove the catheter. In my grogginess and sleepiness I twisted my body up and over to my right side which happened to be the side of the bed that all the cords and tubes were on. It also happened to be the side of my body that all of the five incisions were on, so to get over and up and out of the bed was a pretty painful adventure for me. As I stretched and moaned I sat up and swung my legs over the side of the bed and that was when it happened. That was when I really did it to that poor little, not a tiny person but just young, girl that was helping me to recover and get through the night.

POP! Out came my chest tube. I felt it when it happened. It wasn't a painful sort of thing. It was more like when you put your thumb in your mouth and you flick it against the inside of your cheek as you attempt to make that loud popping sound. Like a cork coming out of a bottle of cabernet sauvignon. The second it happened I knew what had happened and I slowly reached underneath my hospital gown to retrieve the popped-out chest tube. Slowly I pulled it out from underneath my gown and slowly I held it up and showed it to the nurse.

"I think I accidentally sat on this tube." I looked up at her.

"OH NO!" She was freaking out! She literally began to shake all over her entire body. She was in a complete state of panic and she was yelling for help from the other nurses that were in the main desk area of the wing. Many of them came running. I, of course, decided to lay down onto my left side to try and keep my body from immediately vomiting. I felt unbelievably sick and thought for sure I was going to pass out! The nurses got the tube put back in and I apologized profusely for putting them all through such a state of panic. The next morning I awoke to my surgeon standing above me with his hands on his hips.

"I heard you pulled your chest tube out."

"I didn't mean to."

He chuckled and checked to make sure that all of my tubes, cords, beepers and connections were in place and then he told me to try and behave.

And now I'm finally home.

I got through the procedure, the five days stay in the hospital full of wonderful people and now I'm lying in my glorious king size bed in my brand new bedroom, looking out the window over the calm flowing waters that lead into one of the many gorgeous lakes of New Hampshire. And the birds are so incredible. I've seen ducks with red heads, green heads with white rings, white heads, and black heads with large white circles around their eyes. Some of them look like their heads are pointed, while others have the most bulbous round heads which I imagine the sort of heads that alien ducks would have. Sometimes if the timing is perfect I can stand at the window and look down and into the water below just as the smaller red-headed ducks swim by and chase after whatever it is that they want to eat. It's either that or they just love to swim and for some reason that's how they move the quickest. Maybe their feet are too far towards the back of their bodies, like the Loon's. Whatever the case, I love watching them and drifting off to sleep as the curtains blow gently across the top of my king size bed.

And my journey has really just begun. My recovery will take me nearly four months before my body is to the point that I no longer need to take heavy narcotics to get through a day full of pain and so much discomfort that I never would have imagined I'd ever have to go through. And I've had some surgeries before this one; I've had my thyroid removed, a spinal fusion and a C-section for the birth of the twins and a hysterectomy. I do have a bit of experience with pain and recovery after surgery. But nothing that I'd experienced in my life came close to the pain associated with thoracic surgery. Who knew that the lungs are completely covered with nerve endings? I guess it makes sense though as our bodies were really designed to keep us and things away from the most important parts of our bodies. The nerves will scream and tell whoever the intruder is to back off and get the hell away from the things that they are protecting for our very survival; such as lungs and a heart!

Probably the first two months of my recovery from surgery were really nothing more than visits from family and friends, pain killers and sleep. That's about all I remember about it! I remember the first day I gave in to Albert's request to just leave the house and go for a quick ride in our convertible; 'maybe get an ice cream,' he said. Well, the minute the car pulled out of the driveway I knew I'd made a mistake and we quickly turned the car around and got me back into my glorious bed. Just the slightest bump in the road as the car pulled out caused such horrific pain that I couldn't stand it and I just needed to get back into the house, take more pain killers and try to go to sleep. It was a long couple of months, a lot of sleep and a lot of pain killers but eventually I could tolerate a quick jaunt around the corner to get some ice cream with Albert.

The second couple of months I had the luxury of puttering around my new house and actually unpacking our things, decorating rooms and setting up our lives within the house that I truly have come to LOVE! With every day the pain became a bit easier to tolerate. And every day I walked outside with our tiny little solid black Yorki-Poo. I remembered what the incredible nurses had told me to do; 'breathing needs to be a part of your recovery' and 'you need to walk'. So I walked. I walked with my dog along the railroad tracks that border the edge of my new home. I walked and I took pictures of some of the most beautiful sunrises and sunsets that I've ever seen. And I saw some incredible wildlife, which actually surprised me. I never would have imagined that living in a 'downtown' house would still afford me the pleasure of seeing deer, raccoons, skunks, porcupines, a fox and even a coyote. I think the only thing that is left for me to see right in my tiny backyard between the house and the water is a moose and a black bear!

Eventually I went back to the job that I worked to get for more than five years. Back in the building where the snake had continued to devour innocent associates in my absence. Back to the life that I had relocated my entire family for, in the great State of New Hampshire. And really except for the surgery and my rather lengthy medical leave nothing had changed in my life. What ended up being nearly an entire year from the discovery of the 'something's there' to the day I stepped foot back into my store after the medical leave, had in fact just been an interruption. My life around the cancer-project had remained the same. It was as if my life had just stood still and patiently waited for my reinsertion into it.

On the first day of my reinsertion my boss greeted me at the front entrance to the store. He was smiling as he shook my hand and told me how much the team had missed me and how happy he was to see me back to work. And I'm sure that he was completely relieved that I was returning as quickly and as soon as I was physically able to. I was as anxious as he was to get things underway with my new job, in a new place, with a new team. The interruption was not something that had comfortably fit into my plan and my promise to do a good job for him and the company that I work for.

"So what now?" He needed more information. He needed to know if that was it. He needed to have some reassurance that I was actually going to be able to work now that the cancer had been cut from my body.

"Well, the surgery removed the tumors and hopefully that will be exactly the end of it for me. I will have to return to Boston every so often for scans and follow up to make sure that is the case."

"Wow, really?" My boss is surprised. He's relieved but he seems completely surprised. And I understand exactly why he is. Most of the time when you hear of somebody getting cancer it does not amount to a 'just cut it out' sort of procedure. It's a more lengthy process. There's other stuff that has to happen!

"Hopefully! That's the plan at this point! And the great news is that I have the best Oncologist in the world! He's at Dana Farber and he leads in Carcinoid Cancer research. He's sort of studying me because the location of my particular tumors is incredibly rare. I'm lucky to have him as my doctor and if something else happens I'm in good hands."

"What else could happen?" He looks serious now.

I stared at him for a moment and I wasn't really sure how to answer that question. I don't know what else could happen. I don't know what to expect because even the true experts in the cancer fields, including my amazing Oncologist, do not have all of the answers. How can I be expected to answer such a question when I am really a case study of sorts; I'm not one of the experts.

I can tell my boss what I believe will happen! I believe that more will come. I believe that this was too easy and it's never easy when you have to deal with a tragedy that interrupts your life when you least expect it. I can tell him that I'm still sort of pissed off at the whole 'something's there' thing! I can tell him that there are some days that it hits me again and my body slides back into the deep dark stench-filled muddy hand-dug Canterbury well. I can tell him that every time I speak with one of the experts at the Dana Farber hospital I become a zombie again and cock my head to the right as drool drips down my chin. I can tell him that my family is amazing and they support whatever I decide to do with my life. I can tell him that they want me to quit work because they are concerned for my well-being but at the same time they smile at me when I say 'have a good day' as I walk out of the house to start the car and drive back to the store and the team that I manage.

I smiled at my boss and I shook my head.

"Anything could happen. And if anything does…I'll just keep swimming."

The Last Chapter

It's been almost two years since the first cancer chapter began to write itself. Almost two years ago I suddenly had a burning pain when I lifted my right arm and I thought for sure I must have torn ligaments or tendons or something to be causing such extreme discomfort. It was almost two years ago that the call came in from Brad at the Orthopedic Center and he told me that 'something's there!' And then things really began to happen. Almost two years ago I didn't see it coming. I never thought I'd ever be one of those people. The ones that get really sick. The ones that have to face such a curve ball, that they get struck right in the side of the jaw by it rather than just swinging the bat and hitting the freaking thing!

I was diagnosed with a rare form of cancer that is truly considered to be a pink and purple striped zebra of sorts. In fact if you ever see a person wearing a zebra striped ribbon or pin in support of cancer, they are supporting the kind of cancer that I have. I have Carcinoid Cancer. It is a rare type of cancer and makes up for one-percent of all cancers. When the 'Something's there' was discovered we thought that I had a couple of medium sized tumors sort of underneath my armpit but inside of my ribcage; growing within the pleura lining of my right lung. And it was because of these tumors that I underwent a radical surgery during which the outer lining of the pleura was removed. A few months after that, follow up scans revealed that more tumors are actually still inside of me. This was right around the time that I was introduced to one of the best Oncologists in the world who studies Carcinoid Cancer at the Dana Farber Hospital in Boston, Massachusetts.

At this point I have had so many scans and tests that I truly couldn't even guess as to how many. The tumors have metastasized and as of today I have multiple tumors throughout the pleura lining that remains around my right lung, throughout the pleura lining around my left lung, my T7 vertebra, and my left femur. So the 'Something's there!' statement ended up becoming more of a 'You've been invaded!' statement. When all of the locations were discovered my oncologist and I decided that the best course of action was to begin chemotherapy. It no longer makes sense to cut up a body and keep removing parts and pieces when there are quite literally more than twenty locations and some of those locations are chiseling a course right through the largest bone in your body as well as your spine! Time to take a more blanket approach!

The kind of chemotherapy that I've been taking is the kind that they fortunately developed into an oral pill. I didn't need to get a port put into my body and I take the chemotherapy pills within the comfort of my own home. I take the pills five days out of every twenty-eight days. Five days on and twenty-three days off. In other words, every fourth Tuesday I begin taking the drug again. And every fourth Tuesday I also take another six prescriptions in order to better manage the side effects of the drug. The side effects are pretty typical: Nausea, fatigue, dizziness, headaches, diarrhea, constipation, confusion, rectal bleeding, dry skin, rashes and an overall feeling of feeling like shit! I never lost my hair though! In fact my hair has actually grown to be quite long! Since beginning the therapy I've stopped using any heating products or dye on my hair so it's actually done nothing but grow all the way down to the center of my back!

The chemotherapy drug I've been taking is called Temodar and it's also available generically (Temozolomide). I began taking it in March of 2015 and I am getting ready to begin my eleventh round in just three more days from the writing of this chapter. My blood is taken a few days before all scheduled rounds of chemotherapy and so far my labs have been good enough to continue taking the rounds. The plan is to take a full year of the drug, which will mean I have just two more rounds to get through. At that point my body will be given a break because chemotherapy is not something that a person can continue to take forever. At some point we need to recover from the damage being done to the good cells within our bodies. At some point we need to just stop feeling so sick and continue to just breathe.

To date we have yet to discover the primary site for my particular cancer. It MAY be that it all started within the pleura lining around my right lung but that would be extremely rare! It MAY be that it all began within my bones but that would also be extremely rare! More than likely everything began in my lung or in my liver but that has yet to be confirmed; it's just statistically the best guess. And why would any of that matter anyway? Well, apparently knowing where it all began can alter the choice of attack! I guess some cancers are Ninja Warriors and you attack them with sophisticated Ninja moves or you throw spiny metal stars at them or whack them with swords. And then there are other cancers that are Sumo Wrestlers and you need to be bigger and stronger than them so you can push them right out of the ring. And yet still there are cancers that are like heavy weight boxers and if you hit them just right, across the underside of their jaw, they will fall over like a mighty redwood getting chopped down, deep within the California woods. Apparently these different types of cancers respond differently to different types of chemotherapy drugs. However, there are many of us that never know where it all began! So we just deal with what we know as best we can. My Oncologist and I chose to go with proven statistics when picking the type of chemotherapy drug that I would take. Carcinoid cancer does not respond well with chemotherapy but Temodar had a proven track record of eighteen percent.

Last week I had multiple scans. Three different ones in fact. Two of the scans were to look for the primary site that remains a hidden gem within the treasure chest of gems that my body is housing. No luck still. The other scan looked at a soft tissue mass that is nestled between my right lung and the spine. And the GREAT news was/is that although we didn't find the primary site, the scans revealed no growth!

When I first heard 'no growth' I couldn't help but feel disappointed. I thought I was going to hear that the cancer had melted away. I thought when I started taking a drug that was literally killing GOOD cells within my body, that it would at the same time demolish the cells that were BAD. I thought I was going to be one of those people that gets to say 'I'm cancer free!' But I should have remembered that when we started this course of action I was told that Carcinoid Cancer does not respond well to chemotherapy. So actually 'no growth' is an amazing thing! It means that there is nothing new. It means that the tumors are potentially stabilizing.

Now the better news and the theory that I am hanging my hat

on is that once the chemotherapy is stopped and my body is given a break, the cancerous tumors will continue to lay dormant within my body. Sometimes the chemotherapy will actually kill the DNA structure of the cancer cells thereby causing their death! Death meaning that they no longer live, breathe or pulsate! They're still there but they're just empty shells. So I guess that would result with my body housing the tiny cancer corpses for the remainder of my life, which hopefully will be for another forty or so years! I guess that will mean that my body will virtually become a tomb for dead cancer warriors. Rather than burying their bodies on a hillside overlooking a vast meadow of daisies and flying fuzz (because truly they do NOT deserve that), their dead horrific rotting bodies will hide within the deep dark shadows of my organs, bones and pulsating flesh. That will be the BEST news!!! And I'll take it when it happens! I will accept that the cancer will always be within me and I will proudly know that the corpses of the cancerous warriors lie dead within the recesses of my LIVING flesh!

I know everything will be okay. I've always known that everything is going to be okay. Even when I had my melt downs (and there were more than a few of those) I have always found my way back to my heart. My head could not ever lead the way because my head knows nothing about cancer and what to expect. My head had to have conversations with my Oncologist in order to wrap itself around anything having to do with this adventure that I'm on. But I have truly always known within my heart that everything would be okay. My heart has always known that this thing, this cancer, this freaking unforeseen adventure that interrupted my plans was not and will never be my end! It's a pain in my ass but it's not going to be my end.

I'm not sure who 'they' is. I'm not sure who was the first person that ever said, 'they say' but nonetheless I know that 'they' is a true person or entity. And THEY say that when you deal with a tragedy such as divorce, death or getting cancer you go through certain stages. THEY say that the stages follow a certain series of events and mental states and include things such as denial, anger, bargaining, depression and acceptance. And 'they' say that it happens in that order. It didn't happen that way for me though. I'm sure I went through everything that 'they' said I would go through but I'm sure all of my stages were exaggerated, muddled, messy and completely repetitive. My stages if I had to list them were probably closer to something like: Shock, anger, distrust, more anger, rage, confusion, fear, zombification, more anger, maxification, devastation, zombification round two, major rage, exhaustion, more confusion, acceptance, even more rage, confidence and control! I believe we are all different and there is no right or wrong way to get through a life changing event. And I also believe that even if you reach the end of the stages that 'they' say you go through when dealing with a tragedy, the stages have a way of popping back into your life from time to time.

I still turn into a zombie when I'm sitting and listening to my Oncologist talk. I still get really pissed off when out of nowhere I am so dizzy that I have to just sit down and rest. I still cry when I wake in the middle of the night to find myself slipping back through the stench filled mud within the hand-dug Canterbury well. In my experience the stages are part of the journey and as long as the journey continues so will the reappearance of the stages.

My journey is an ongoing mystery. It's a journey that I never thought I'd be taking and it's a journey that I didn't plan out, buy plane tickets for, rent a hotel room for or invite friends and family to come and meet me along the way. I can't for the life of me figure out who did it in the ballroom and with what weapon but I will continue to try and make sense of it all. Along my journey I am meeting people that are truly incredible and they should truly be an inspiration for an entire generation because they are the ones that feed me and many others the directions along the path. They are like the GPS's for those of us that are on this cancer journey. They are the ones speaking in the background when we are lost in the dark and struggling to find our focus. They are the ones that say 'turn left up ahead'.

I consider myself to be so lucky. I am lucky that the 'something's there' was even discovered. I am lucky that the kind of cancer I have is a slow growing cancer. It might have already spread throughout my body and set up little colonies of additional cancer friends and family but it moves slowly. The slower it moves, the more time the ones that guide me have to try and destroy the little cancer warriors. I am so lucky to have one of the best Oncologists in the world that is trying to figure out, not only a solution for me, but multiple solutions for the masses of people that also received a call that told them 'something's there'!

Behind all of my incredible luck stands my family. They are the ones that have taken every step of this journey with me. They walked along the twisting winding paths through the dark and dangerous forest with me even though they were terrified. They are the ones that held my head above the water as I struggled to swim against the monstrous waves in the center of the deepest ocean. They are the ones that reached beneath the mud and stretched with all of their might to grab hold of my body and hoist me up and away from the horrific stench within the hand-dug Canterbury well. They are the ones that tell me to listen to my heart because it knows that I will be okay.

I am still on my journey and I always will be. The journey will never be over. And that's okay with me because if it were I would have written a different book and the story would have ended long ago. My book is just my story and it is really only the first chapter. I'm excited to still be on this journey because it is completely full of mystery, love, discoveries and dreams. A journey is really just the act of moving from one place to another and a journey is what each and every one of us is on. We are all headed in the same direction and the only difference between us is what we do along the way. What we do along the way is what truly defines who we are. What we do along the way is what gets us to the destination.

Not… The End

www.ingramcontent.com/pod-product-compliance
Lightning Source LLC
Chambersburg PA
CBHW070108290526
45789CB00005B/1970